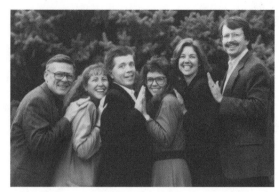

Our "Compacted" Compact Clinicals Team

Dear Valued Customer,

WELCOME to Compact Clinicals. We are committed to bringing mental health professionals up-to-date diagnostic and treatment information in a compact, timesaving, and easy-to-read format. Our line of books provides current, thorough reviews of assessment and treatment strategies for mental disorders.

We've "compacted" complete information for diagnosing each disorder and comparing how different theoretical orientations approach treatment. Our books use nonacademic language, real-world examples, and well-defined terminology.

Enjoy this and other timesaving books from Compact Clinicals.

Sincerely,

Melanie Dean, Ph.D.
President

Compact Clinicals Line of Books

Compact Clinicals currently offers these condensed reviews for professionals:

For Clinicians

Attention Deficit Hyperactivity Disorder
The latest assessment and treatment strategies

C. Keith Conners, Ph.D.

Bipolar Disorder
The latest assessment and treatment strategies

Trisha Suppes M.D., Ph.D., and Ellen B. Dennehy, Ph.D.

Borderline Personality Disorder
The latest assessment and treatment strategies

Melanie Dean, Ph.D.

Conduct Disorders
The latest assessment and treatment strategies

J. Mark Eddy, Ph.D.

Depression in Adults
The latest assessment and treatment strategies

Anton Tolman, Ph.D.

Obsessive Compulsive Disorder
The latest assessment and treatment strategies

Gail Steketee, Ph.D., and Teresa Pigot, M.D.

Post-Traumatic and Acute Stress Disorders
The latest assessment and treatment strategies

Matthew Friedman, M.D., Ph.D.

For Physicians

Bipolar Disorder: Treatment and Management
Trisha Suppes, M.D., Ph.D., and Paul E. Keck, Jr., M.D.

Bipolar Disorder

The latest assessment and treatment strategies

Trisha Suppes, M.D., Ph.D.

Ellen B. Dennehy, Ph.D.

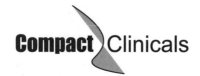

Compact Clinicals

This book is intended for use by properly trained and licensed mental health professionals, who already possess a solid education in psychological theory, research, and treatment. This book is in no way intended to replace or supplement such training and education, nor is it to be used as the sole basis for any decision regarding treatment. It is merely intended to be used by such trained and educated professionals as a review and resource guide when considering how to best treat an adult with bipolar disorder.

Bipolar Disorder

The latest assessment and treatment strategies

by

Trisha Suppes, M.D., Ph.D., and Ellen B. Dennehy, Ph.D.

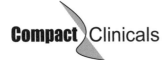

Published by: Compact Clinicals
7205 NW Waukomis Dr., Suite A
Kansas City, MO 64151
816-587-0044

©2005 Dean Psych Press Corp. d/b/a Compact Clinicals

Medical Editing: Kathi Whitman, In Credible English, Inc.,®
Kansas City, Missouri

Book Design: Coleridge Design, Kansas City, Missouri

Library of Congress Cataloging in Publication data:

Suppes, Trisha
Bipolar disorder : the latest assessment and treatment strategies / by
Trisha Suppes, Ellen Dennehy
     p.   cm.
  Includes bibliographical references and index.
  ISBN 1-887537-25-2
  1. Manic-depressive illness. 2. Manic-depressive illness–Treatment.
I. Dennehy, Ellen, 1968- II. Title.
  RC516.S864 2005
  616.89'5–dc22
       2005002098

10 9 8 7 6 5 4 3 2

Read Me First

As a mental health professional, often the information you need can only be obtained after countless hours of reading or library research. If your schedule precludes this time commitment, Compact Clinicals is the answer.

Our books are practitioner oriented with easy-to-read treatment descriptions and examples. Compact Clinicals books are written in a nonacademic style. Our books are formatted to make the first reading, as well as ongoing reference, quick and easy. You will find:

▶ **Anecdotes** — Each chapter contains a fictionalized account that personalizes the disorder entitled, "From the Patient's Perspective."

▶ **Sidebars** — Narrow columns on the outside of each page highlight important information, preview upcoming sections or concepts, and define terms used in the text.

▶ **Definitions** — Terms are defined in the sidebars where they originally appear in the text and in an alphabetical glossary on pages 93 through 96.

▶ **References** — Numbered references appear in the text following information from that source. Full references appear on pages 97 through 108.

▶ **Case Examples** — Our examples illustrate typical adult client comments or conversational exchanges that help clarify different treatment approaches. Identifying information in the examples (e.g., the individual's real name, profession, age, and/or location) has been changed to protect the confidentiality of those clients discussed in case examples.

▶ **Key Concepts** — At the end of each chapter, we include a review list of key concepts from that chapter. Use these lists for ongoing quick reference as well as for reviewing what you learned from reading the chapter.

Contents

Chapter 3: Biological Treatment of Bipolar Disorder 25

Chapter One:
General Information about Bipolar Disorder

This chapter answers the following:

▶ **What is Bipolar Disorder?** — This section defines the disorder, introduces possible causes, and presents the four categories of diagnoses associated with the disorder.

▶ **How Does the Disorder Affect Patients' Lives?** — This section covers the impacts of mania, hypomania, depression, and mixed episodes on patients' lives.

▶ **How Common is Bipolar Disorder?** — This section gives prevalence rates for the U.S. and Europe.

▶ **What is the Likelihood of Recovery?** — This section discusses the importance of treatment plan compliance in reducing symptoms of the disorder.

F OR those with bipolar disorder, as well as for their families and friends, life is an unpredictable and debilitating series of emotional highs and lows. Often referred to in the past as manic-depression, bipolar disorder represents a biological condition characterized by rapid mood swings. A manic episode brings on euphoria, recklessness, compromised financial security, and relationship problems. When the pendulum swings to a depressive episode, there is extreme hopelessness and listlessness.

Originally, mania was a nonspecific term for madness, and melancholia was a type of "madness" characterized by a withdrawn and quiet demeanor.

Today, over 2,000,000 American adults suffer from bipolar disorder. The first episodes typically appear in adolescence or early adulthood when life stresses are at their greatest. For women, bipolar disorder may be triggered by childbirth or menopause.

Although there is no single, documented cause or known cure for bipolar disorder, medications and other therapies can help manage the symptoms. Without treatment, the disorder can worsen, with manic episodes becoming more frequent, intense, and characterized by more psychotic behavior.

What is Bipolar Disorder?

"Mania" and "melancholia" — ancient terms for two, distinct mood changes — characterize the disorder today referred to as bipolar disorder. Historically, 19th century physicians recognized alternating episodes of *mania* and *depression* as distinct disorders, and, by the early 1900s, bipolar disorder was distinguished from schizophrenia. In 1952, the first edition of the Diagnostic and Statistical Manual of Mental Disorders presented an early conceptualization of the disorder.[1]

mania — a mood state characterized by an elevated or irritable mood, decreased sleep, high energy, impulsive behavior, and increased goal-directed behavior

depression — a mood state characterized by sadness or irritability, low energy, thoughts of death and suicide, and lack of interest in previously enjoyed activities

impulsivity — taking action with limited thought to consequences

hypomania — a mood state characterized by increased energy, excitement, and feelings of euphoria that do not meet the diagnostic criteria for a full manic episode

dysphoric hypomania — a mood state characterized by increased energy and symptoms of depression that do not meet full criteria for depression

psychotic — extreme impairment of a person's ability to think clearly, perceive things accurately, respond emotionally, communicate effectively, understand reality, and behave appropriately

PET imaging — technology that uses positron-labeled molecules and an oxygen blood flow tracer to develop images of brain activity versus the structural images provided by MRI

euthymia — normal range of mood, no evidence of mania, hypomania, or depression

Bipolar disorder is a mood disorder for which the exact cause is unknown. It is characterized by significant swings between mania and depression, as well as changes in sleep patterns, energy, activity, attention, and *impulsivity*. Although there are many variations of mood patterns and severity that a person with bipolar disorder might experience, he or she generally experiences periods of mania, *hypomania,* or *dysphoric hypomania*, and major depressive episodes. Patients may also experience *psychotic* symptoms when manic or depressed.

Through *PET imaging,* which detects differences in the brain activity of people who are depressed or manic compared to those experiencing a normal mood state, researchers are gaining a better understanding of the causes of bipolar disorder. As a result, experts now believe that a dysregulation (not unlike an epileptic seizure) occurs in the brain cells regulating emotions, circadian rhythms, and behaviors, thus causing bipolar symptoms.[2]

One challenging feature of bipolar disorder is that patients' experiences of the illness can vary tremendously, with some patients suffering depression followed by hypomania, and others mania followed by depression. Some move quickly from episode to episode, with virtually no period of mood stability (*euthymia*) in between significant ups and downs. Others may be relatively stable between discrete episodes of mania or depression for longer periods. Defining an individual's characteristic pattern can impact choice of treatments.

The graph in figure 1.1, on the next page, illustrates these varying patterns in two patients: Sue, a 55-year-old secretary and John, a 28-year-old, unemployed construction worker.

Most patients with bipolar disorder first experience symptoms before age 25, with the average age of onset around 20.[3] However, the average time from symptom onset to correct diagnosis is often eight to nine years. This is due to bipolar symptoms being difficult to recognize and developing gradually, rather than all at once, and being difficult to recognize.[4, 5]

A person's first significant episode is usually associated with stressful life events, such as beginning a new job, going to college, getting married, or having a child.

Over time, the duration of "well" periods between mood episodes can decrease in some individuals, leading to a more chronic, severe course with more episodes of mania or depression. Others may start out experiencing one episode per year and continue at this frequency. Studies conducted in the early 1900s (before medication treatment) indicate that some patients experienced less time between episodes as they aged. For example, in the early days of their illness, the characteristic course for one individual might have been three to four years between episodes; however, as they aged, they might have experienced 12–18 months between mood episodes. This is still the course of the illness for some patients, who have a range of presentations and course of illness patterns. However, others develop chronic ongoing symptoms, with few days of relatively symptom-free function between acute episodes. Evidence suggests that those who experience more episodes before treatment begins may develop greater resistance to treatment, making early detection and intervention important.[6]

An area of research and debate revolves around a growing body of literature, broadening bipolar disorder diagnostic criteria to include a spectrum of mood manifestations not meeting criteria for BD-I, BD-II, or BD-NOS. For example, some see "bipolarity" as a dimensional illness continuous from BD-I through entities not currently categorized by DSM-IV(TR) (e.g., borderline bipolar, soft bipolar, and affective temperaments, such as hyperthymic, cyclothymic, dysthymic, irritable) and in-between disorders (e.g., bipolar III).[7-9] Further research is needed to determine the link between this interface of symptoms and "temperament" and subsequent implications for illness course and treatment.

Chapters three and four detail appropriate treatment choices for varied symptom patterns.

Figure 1.1   Individual Characteristic Patterns

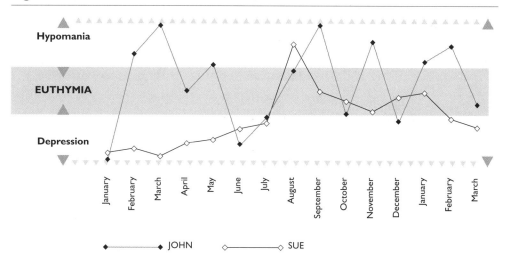

How Does the Disorder Affect Patients' Lives?

Those with bipolar disorder typically find that their quality of life and ability to function changes, even with adequate treatment and symptom remission.[10–13]

Specific Impacts of Mania

circadian rhythms — the daily regulation of sleep-wake cycles and activity-to-activity patterns

Typically, those experiencing a **manic episode** find they sleep less or not at all due to a disruption in their *circadian rhythms*. Despite this, they sustain high energy levels (e.g., a person in a full manic episode may feel little or no need for sleep, exercise several hours daily, and have "boundless" energy for new projects). However, this energy may not be focused in a productive fashion, and the patient may go for many days without sleeping. In fact, patients in the 19th century (prior to medication treatment) would sometimes die from manic episodes due to lack of sleep and neglecting to eat or drink water.

grandiosity — exaggerated belief or claims of one's importance or identity; manifested as delusions of great wealth, power, or fame when of psychotic proportions

Classic mania is also associated with *grandiosity* and behavior that family and friends recognize as atypical for the individual, such as: spending sprees, promiscuity, alcohol or drug abuse, or other impulsive, potentially risky behavior. Patients with bipolar disorder may neither recognize their symptoms nor, as mania worsens, the consequences of their risky behavior because of the confusion and loss of contact with reality that occurs when the disorder remains untreated. Mania can profoundly disrupt an individual's life, often leading to joblessness, financial instability, and damaged family relationships.

Over 50 percent of those with bipolar disorder will experience a lifetime prevalence of alcohol and/or substance abuse or dependence.[17] Many bipolar patients also may suffer from eating disorders and impulse control problems.[15]

The Impacts of Bipolar Disorder and Substance Abuse

In general, impacts of bipolar disorder may be more serious when associated with other disorders, such as alcohol and drug abuse.[14, 15] Compared to the general population, men and women with bipolar disorder are four times and eight times, respectively, more likely to become alcoholic.[16]

Substance abuse may have a cumulative impact on the brain, affecting course and treatment response. For example, one study found that a history of substance abuse further complicates the course of bipolar disorder and has significant treatment implications, such as lower rates of remission and poor response to lithium.[18] In addition, substance use is associated with poor treatment compliance.[19] Thus, patients must be cautioned against substance abuse, an important clinical point, given research that finds a greater than 50 percent lifetime prevalence of substance abuse (including alcohol) among patients with bipolar disorder.[17]

Specific Impacts of Hypomania

Those experiencing **hypomania** feel "on top of the world," able to accomplish anything, sociable, creative, and invigorated. Thus, these symptoms are rarely reported as patients perceive them as positive and beneficial. Hypomania typically progresses to mania in patients with bipolar I disorder and is (by definition) a change from usual functioning observed by others. While not as severe as mania, hypomania makes a patient more prone to making impulsive decisions, which can have lasting consequences. The majority of patients experiencing hypomania are in an unstable mood state, often progressing to mania or depression.

Many patients will experience a combination of hypomania and depression, also termed "mixed hypomania."

Specific Impacts of Depression

Depression often impacts people's sleeping and eating habits, causing some to:

▶ Wake up feeling tired from being up and down all night and waking earlier than usual

▶ Sleep far more than normal

▶ Have little or no appetite

▶ Gain weight from overeating

▶ Find food unsatisfying or unappealing

Depressed people often have trouble concentrating, remembering, and making decisions. They may be unable to concentrate on a television program or book, decide what to wear, or whether to renew a subscription, feeling that these decisions are overwhelming or exhausting. Persons with depression report very low self-esteem, and often dwell on their negative qualities, failings, or losses. They also report feelings of hopelessness: a belief that nothing will ever improve; exaggerated pessimism.

At least 75 percent of suicides among those with bipolar disorder occur when these patients are experiencing either depressed or mixed episodes.[20] Chapter two includes a section on assessing suicide risk (pages 20 to 21).

From the Patient's Perspective

I can't believe how productive I am! Like today: it's 2:15 am, and I am still going strong. Just finished buying some new Christmas decorations online, started cleaning the house, fixed the kids' lunches for the week. Next, I'm going to tackle the office paperwork. I even worked out! I hope this extra energy lasts; I don't know what I did to deserve this, but I feel great. I feel very competent, happy, and productive; it sure feels better than the "down-in-the-dumps" winter I had.

Specific Impacts of Mixed Episodes

Additionally, many patients experience a mix of symptoms, with depressive symptoms either occurring simultaneously or within a short time of hypomanic or manic symptoms. For example, a patient could be very irritable with a depressed mood and also feel very energized and make impulsive decisions. Patients may also experience mixed symptoms without meeting full criteria for either mania or depression.

For information on assessing suicide risk, see pages 20–21.

Bipolar disorder may also be accompanied by a high risk for self-injury and suicide when symptoms persist untreated, patients fail to take medications as prescribed, or when patients experience a limited response to treatment.[21, 22]

How Common is Bipolar Disorder?

The latest estimates of bipolar disorder prevalence in the U.S. indicate that 1.5 percent of the population suffer from the disorder.[20] However, about 30 percent of people with the illness have either been diagnosed and are not receiving treatment, are undiagnosed, or have been diagnosed in error — usually as having major depressive disorder alone. In Europe, where a broader definition of the illness doesn't require the same duration criteria for hypomanic or depressive symptoms, estimates are higher — totaling as much as five percent of the population.[23]

Chapter three reviews the biological bases of bipolar disorder in detail.

Additionally, genetic and environmental factors may either cause or intensify this dysregulation. Possible environmental factors include substance abuse, medical problems (e.g., thyroid fluctuation), stressful life events, and lifestyles that prohibit regulated sleep-wake cycles. Research also demonstrates that genetics may be a factor in bipolar disorder.[24, 25]

What is the Likelihood of Recovery?

Bipolar disorder is a lifelong, recurrent illness. Once diagnosed, continued consultation and treatment is necessary to reduce symptoms. Treatment commonly involves taking one or more medications. Patients can improve their prognosis by:

- ▶ Cooperating with health care professionals and their treatment plan
- ▶ Taking medications as directed
- ▶ Detecting changes in symptoms early by monitoring their moods and behaviors related to bipolar disorder
- ▶ Enhancing brain chemistry by making healthy diet and exercise choices

Sudden discontinuation of prescribed medications can worsen bipolar disorder by reducing the patient's response to medication in the future and/or increasing the frequency of episodes.

Those with untreated bipolar disorder are typically unstable, experiencing uncomfortable and unpredictable mood states as well as changes in energy, sleep, and behavior. Even when treated, medications may have to be adjusted as patients face new episodes or breakthrough symptoms. However, with effective medication treatment, many patients experience a reduction or remission in symptoms.

This book is intended for the professional in the field. Clinicians working with patients with bipolar disorder will find information to supplement their work, as follows:

- ▶ **Chapter two** covers assessment and diagnostic techniques as well as how to differentiate between bipolar disorder and other disorders with similar symptoms.
- ▶ **Chapter three** addresses the biological origins of the disorder as well as pharmacological and other biologically based treatment approaches.
- ▶ **Chapter four** covers psychosocial treatment approaches used in conjunction with medication therapy.
- ▶ **Appendix A** presents the DSM-IV (TR) criteria for bipolar disorder.
- ▶ **Appendix B** includes detailed information on assessment tools listed in chapter two.
- ▶ **Appendix C** includes a sample log from the Life Chart, a self-report method for documenting bipolar symptoms.

Key Concepts for Chapter One:

1. Bipolar disorder is a mood disorder that appears to be caused by a dysregulation in brain chemistry, which can be accentuated by genetics and environmental factors.

2. Bipolar disorder is characterized by mood swings that vary from one patient to another in duration, intensity, order of occurrence, and length of symptom-free period between episodes.

3. When symptoms persist untreated, medication compliance is low, or when there is limited response to treatment, patients with bipolar disorder may have a high risk for self-injury and suicide.

4. Patients often fail to recognize manic symptoms, especially when mania worsens as they become confused and lose contact with reality. Also, patients with hypomanic symptoms may fail to report these symptoms as they perceive them to be positive and beneficial.

5. There is a strong association between bipolar disorder and alcohol and/or substance abuse or dependence, a history of either signifying a potentially more severe course of illness and less response to treatment.

6. Bipolar disorder is a lifelong, recurrent illness that can be treated with medications so that patients can enjoy a more stable lifestyle and relationships.

Chapter Two:
Diagnosing and Assessing Bipolar Disorder

This chapter answers the following:

▶ **What are the Typical Symptoms of Bipolar Disorder?** — This section reviews the typical symptoms of mania, hypomania, and depression.

▶ **What are the Criteria for Diagnosing Bipolar Disorder?** — This section presents the DSM-IV (TR) criteria for making a diagnosis as well as diagnostic clarifiers.

▶ **What Tools Exist for Diagnosing Bipolar Disorder?** — This section offers direction on conducting medical assessments and clinical interviews as well as using clinician- and self-rated assessment tools.

▶ **What Differentiates Bipolar Disorder from Other Disorders?** — This section reviews the various physiological and psychological disorders that may be difficult to distinguish from bipolar diagnoses or coexist with bipolar disorder.

▶ **How does Bipolar Disorder Present in Children and Adolescents?** — This section overviews issues related to diagnosing and treating bipolar disorder for these age groups.

ASSESSING bipolar disorder involves identifying the patient's range of episodes, including depression, mania or hypomania, and dysphoric or *mixed episodes.* Other factors that help specify the diagnosis include *rapid cycling* and presence of psychosis.

Patients who present for treatment may not reveal all the dimensions of their mood fluctuations; thus, thorough assessment is critical to detect bipolar disorder. In particular, this may occur because of lack of insight; lack of knowledge, and thus failure to recognize symptoms; or desire not to take medications. For example, research demonstrates that many patients seek help while in a depressive episode, and may not spontaneously volunteer information regarding past episodes of hypomania or mania.[23, 26, 27] It is critical that clinicians ask specifically about these types of mood symptoms when first evaluating a depressed patient.

mixed episodes — periods during which symptoms of a manic and a depressive episode are present at the same time

rapid cycling — four or more manic, hypomanic, or depressive episodes in any 12-month period

What are the Typical Symptoms of Bipolar Disorder?

Although the term "typical" may be a misnomer for peoples' experiences with bipolar disorder (in terms of duration of episodes and duration of non-symptomatic periods between episodes), the symptoms of mania, hypomania, and depression are recognizable and similar from patient to patient.

"Dysphoria" derives from a Greek word meaning "distress" or "hard to bear," and is used by the psychiatric and medical community as a diagnostic term; generally referring to subthreshold depression that doesn't meet full criteria for a major depressive episode.

Figure 2.1, on the next page, provides an overview of manic and depressive symptoms. Hypomania is not listed as it is different from mania only in terms of not meeting full diagnostic criteria.

Recognizing Symptoms of Mania

Manic symptoms can appear as:

> ▶ **A highly excited, energetic mood state** — Feeling "on top of the world" and able to achieve anything despite a decreased ability to complete necessary tasks or tend to daily functions. Those with mania feel they need very little sleep or rest. They may spend excessively, participate in indiscriminate social/sexual interactions, or act impulsively. While the manic individual may feel happy and expansive, friends and family will recognize their behavior as excessive, and may refer the person for treatment. Untreated, mania will worsen, with moods becoming more elevated or irritable, behavior more unpredictable, and judgment more impaired. They're often unaware of the consequences of extreme behavior, due to confusion, disorientation, and loss of contact with reality.

> ▶ **An irritable, excited mood** — Moods fluctuate between euphoria and irritability, all charged by excessive energy, restlessness, and agitation. Similar to classic mania, the patient will have a subjective sense of racing thoughts and, while initiating many projects, will finish few.

delusions — false, fixed, odd, or unusual beliefs about external reality that are not ordinarily accepted by other members of the person's culture or subculture, yet are firmly sustained despite clear evidence to the contrary

When manic, some patients experience symptoms of psychosis (including *delusions* and *hallucinations*), indicating being out of touch with reality in certain important ways.

A **manic episode** is defined by a distinct period of persistently elevated, expansive, or irritable mood **lasting at least one week** (or less if hospitalization is required). The mood is also accompanied by additional symptoms, such as those highlighted above.

hallucinations — sensory perceptions (seeing, hearing, feeling, and smelling) in the absence of an outside stimulus

Recognizing Symptoms of Hypomania

Hypomania resembles mania, but does not meet full criteria for a manic episode and is rarely reported for psychiatric intervention, as the person perceives the experience as positive. Hypomanic individuals report feeling on top of things, productive, sociable, and self-confident. They feel excited, energized, creative, active, intelligent, and sometimes, more sexual. They may say that they feel better than at any other time in their lives, and fail to recognize errors in judgment, neglect of everyday duties, or other subtle lapses in functioning. They cannot understand why anyone would call their experience abnormal or part of a disorder.

While the above describes a pure hypomanic episode, many patients (particularly women) will experience mixed symptoms when hypomanic, perhaps having increased irritability, anger, or sadness in conjunction with extra physical and mental energy.[28]

Figure 2.1   Overview of Manic and Depressive Symptoms*

Symptoms of Mania	Symptoms of Depression
• Increased physical and mental activity/energy	• Prolonged sadness or unexplained crying spells
• Heightened mood, exaggerated optimism, and self-confidence	• Significant changes in appetite and sleep patterns
• Excessive irritability, aggressive behavior	• Irritability, anger, worry, agitation, anxiety
• Decreased need for sleep without feeling fatigued	• Pessimism, indifference
• Ambitious or grandiose plans, inflated sense of self-importance	• Loss of energy, persistent lethargy
• Increased or more rapid speech than normal	• Feelings of guilt, worthlessness
• More thoughts than normal, racing thoughts, flight of ideas	• Inability to concentrate, indecisiveness
• Impulsiveness, poor judgment, distractibility	• Inability to take pleasure in former interests, social withdrawal
• Reckless behavior	• Unexplained aches and pains
• Increased sexual interest and/or activity	• Recurring thoughts of death or suicide
• In severe cases, delusions and hallucinations	

*Hypomania is similar to mania except symptoms do not meet full criteria.

Because of this perception, one of the criteria for diagnosing hypomania is a change of state **observable by others.** This noticeable change of state can be best verified by talking with family members or close associates who can comment on previous behavior.

A **hypomanic episode** is defined by a distinct period of persistently elevated, expansive, or irritable mood **lasting at least four days**. The mood is also accompanied by additional symptoms: inflated self-esteem or grandiosity, a decreased need for sleep, pressured speech, flight of ideas, distractibility, increased involvement in goal-directed activities or psychomotor agitation, and excessive involvement in pleasurable and high-risk activities.

Feedback from family and friends helps the clinician distinguish between abnormal elevations of mood and the person's baseline levels of energy, goal-directed behavior, and personality.

Recognizing Symptoms of Depression

A **major depressive episode** is characterized by depressed mood or loss of interest or pleasure in previously enjoyed activities for a period of at least two weeks. Additionally, the individual may experience some or all of the following:

- ▶ Increased or decreased need for sleep
- ▶ Increased or decreased appetite
- ▶ Loss of energy
- ▶ Difficulty initiating action/behavior
- ▶ Diminished ability to concentrate
- ▶ Social withdrawal
- ▶ Feelings of worthlessness
- ▶ Thoughts of suicide or death

See pages 20–21 for a discussion of suicide assessment.

In children and adolescents, the predominant mood may be irritable rather than sad, accompanied by additional symptoms from the list above.

When they are depressed, people with bipolar disorder are often in a profoundly sad, irritable, or "numb" mood. They may report that life is totally without pleasure and not worth living, despite acknowledging positive things that "should" help them feel happy or satisfied. During depression, people lose interest and enjoyment in their usual activities, including basic pleasures, such as eating and sex.

Core depression symptoms are changes in sleeping and eating habits. Many find it difficult to fall asleep, waking up several times each night and earlier in the morning than desired. About 20 percent of depressed people sleep more than they normally do. In all cases, people experiencing depression awaken without feeling rested. Changes in appetite can be determined by a corresponding weight loss or an increase in appetite, without necessarily feeling the food they eat is satisfying or appealing.

Untreated, lengthy periods of severe depression can lead to thoughts about or actual attempts to commit suicide, making treatment particularly critical for those with bipolar disorder.

Persons with depression often have difficulty with concentration, memory, and decision-making. There is impairment in the person's social and/or occupational functioning.

Recognizing a Mixed Episode

A **mixed episode** is characterized by a period of at least one week in which the criteria are met both for a manic episode and for a major depressive episode nearly every day. The individual may experience rapidly alternating moods (sadness, irritability, euphoria) accompanied by symptoms of a manic episode and a major depressive episode.

What are the Criteria for Diagnosing Bipolar Disorder?

The potential diagnoses for someone experiencing alternating mood states include:[20]

Individuals with BD-I must meet criteria for at least one manic or mixed episode in their lifetime.

- ▶ **Bipolar I Disorder (BD-I)** — Patients meet the criteria for **full manic episodes;** most patients experience depressive episodes as well.
- ▶ **Bipolar II Disorder (BD-II)** — Patients experience episodes of **hypomania** and **depression**.
- ▶ **Cyclothymic Disorder** — Patients experience numerous periods of both **hypomanic** and **depressive** symptoms over a two-year period without meeting criteria for full episodes of either.

See appendix A for a reprint of corresponding DSM-IV (TR) criteria.

- ▶ **Bipolar Disorder Not Otherwise Specified (BD-NOS)** — Patients have cyclic moods and other symptoms consistent with bipolar disorder, but do not meet the criteria for any of the other three diagnoses.

Figure 2.2, below, indicates episode types (major depressive, manic, hypomanic, or mixed) that are characteristic for each diagnosis along with a summary of DSM-IV(TR) criteria. The term, "subthreshold symptoms," indicates that the symptoms are not strong enough to meet DSM criteria for a full mood episode. Page 14 also features a summary of the disorder's diagnostic *specifiers*.

specifiers — DSM-IV-defined categories for specific symptoms that may occur with bipolar disorder such as psychotic or atypical symptoms

Figure 2.2 Linking Bipolar Diagnostic Criteria with Depressive, Manic, Hypomanic, and Mixed Episodes

Episodes Associated with Bipolar Disorder	BD-I	BD-II	Cyclo-thymia	Bipolar Disorder NOS
Major Depressive Episode Characteristics • Depressed mood • At least two weeks' duration • Loss of interest or pleasure • Irritable mood rather than sad (in children) • Changes in appetite, weight, sleep, or psychomotor activity • Decreased energy • Feelings of worthlessness or guilt • Difficulty concentrating or making decisions • Recurrent thoughts of death or suicide			Subthreshold Symptoms	Subthreshold Symptoms
Manic Episode Characteristics • Persistently elevated, expansive, or irritable mood • At least one week's duration (or less if hospitalization is required) • Inflated self-esteem or grandiosity • Decreased need for sleep • Pressured speech • Flight of ideas • Distractibility • Increased involvement in goal-directed activities or psychomotor agitation • Excessive involvement in pleasurable and high-risk activities				
Hypomanic Episode Characteristics • Persistently elevated, expansive, or irritable mood • At least four days' duration • Inflated self-esteem or grandiosity • Decreased need for sleep • Pressured speech • Flight of ideas • Distractibility • Increased involvement in goal-directed activities or psychomotor agitation • Excessive involvement in pleasurable and high-risk activities				Subthreshold Symptoms
Mixed Episode Characteristics • Criteria met both for a manic episode and for a major depressive episode nearly every day • Rapidly alternating moods (sadness, irritability, euphoria) accompanied by symptoms of a manic episode and a major depressive episode				

Diagnostic Specifiers for Bipolar I Disorder and Bipolar II Disorder

DSM-IV (TR) explicitly endorses more detailed specifiers for bipolar disorder. These specifiers impact the treatment response and illness course for many patients.

For manic and depressive episodes, specifiers of the current clinical status and/or features include:

▶ Mild, moderate, severe symptoms without psychotic features/severe with psychotic features

▶ Chronic

▶ With *catatonic features*

▶ With *melancholic features*

▶ With *atypical features*

▶ With postpartum onset

During a manic episode, about half of all patients will experience psychotic symptoms. These symptoms in bipolar disorder are often indistinguishable from psychotic symptoms experienced by patients with schizophrenia, including delusions, hallucinations, *tangentiality*, *derailment*, and other signs of cognitive disorganization.

Other Diagnostic Specifiers

In addition to the above specifiers, for patients who are **not currently** in a manic, hypomanic, or depressed state, specify if they are in partial or full remission. For all bipolar disorder diagnoses, specify:

▶ Longitudinal course (with or without inter-episode recovery)

▶ With *seasonal pattern*

▶ With rapid cycling

More common in women than in men, rapid cycling is specified when a person has experienced four or more distinct episodes in the past year. Additionally, growing evidence exists that those with rapid cycling are more treatment resistant.[29-35] In some cases, persons with rapid cycling may experience chronic and persistent symptoms of differing intensity, with little to no intermittent periods of euthymia. The term, "dysphoric mania/hypomania episode," is used to describe when criteria are met for mania or hypomania, but there are either too few depressive symptoms or insufficient duration of these symptoms to meet criteria for a mixed episode.

---

catatonic features — clinical features characterized by marked psychomotor disturbance that may involve immobility, excessive motor activity, extreme negativism, inability or refusal to speak, peculiar voluntary movements or speech

melancholic features — loss of interest or pleasure in all, or almost all activities, and lack of reactivity to usually pleasurable stimuli

atypical features — mood reactivity and at least two of the following: increased appetite or weight gain, excessive sleep, the sensation that your limbs are too heavy to move, and a long-standing pattern of sensitivity to perceived interpersonal rejection

tangentiality — speech characterized by giving unrelated answers to direct questions and frequently changing the topic

derailment — quality of speech characterized by loose associations or an inability to stay on topic; sequential connection between ideas, which are difficult or impossible to follow because the person wanders to relatively or totally unrelated subjects

seasonal pattern — onset and remission of mood episodes occur at characteristic times of the year

What Tools Exist for Diagnosing Bipolar Disorder?

There is no simple diagnostic tool, such as a blood test, to assess for the presence of bipolar disorder. Trained mental health providers conduct clinical interviews and may administer self-report or clinician-rated scales to assess for symptom presence and severity.

This section reviews medical assessment and clinical interviewing (including collecting family psychiatric history) and lists symptom scales used for evaluation — clinician-administered, self-report, and general psychiatric tools. Appendix B presents detailed information on each of the symptom evaluation scales listed in this chapter.

Conducting a Medical Assessment

Since bipolar disorder is a clinical syndrome caused by brain dysfunction, it is important to rule out physiological causes for the symptoms. The DSM-IV (TR) recognizes the potential of medical problems causing clinical symptoms under the diagnosis, "Mood Disorder due to a General Medical Condition."

Some physiological causes to consider are:

▶ **Embolic stroke**, which occurs typically in an elderly individual. For example, parietal lobe strokes have been implicated in both the development of depression and mania for some individuals. The parietal lobe is the brain lobe sitting behind the frontal cortex on each side of the midline.

▶ **Thyroid conditions** include **hyperthyroidism** (an excess of thyroid hormone), which can cause manic-like symptoms, or **hypothyroidism** (decreased thyroid

From the Patient's Perspective

My boss called me in today and was concerned that my work didn't seem to be as complete as a month or two ago. My co-workers are also complaining that I don't follow through on team projects these days. I know something is strange since I only sleep four hours a night. It's just so nice to have all this energy! When the credit card bill came today, my husband went through the roof; $700 in online purchases just in the last week. Maybe I should see a psychiatrist again, just to get everyone off my back.

hormone), which can cause depression-like symptoms. Blood tests will indicate changes in hormone levels.

Both conditions are associated with physical symptoms not usually observed in patients with bipolar disorder (e.g., elevated heart rate and blood pressure in hyperthyroidism and sensitivity to temperature change as well as skin bruises and tears in hypothyroidism).

▶ **Temporal lobe epilepsy**, which is associated with many of the same symptoms that can be seen in bipolar disorder — no coincidence since one of the main brain structures implicated in bipolar disorder is the brain's temporal lobe.

▶ **Neoplastic or cancer syndromes**, which have also been associated with some patients' change in usual presentation and development of bipolar-like symptoms.

Past history of head injuries should always be part of a medical assessment for bipolar disorder because head injury in and of itself can either cause or aggravate bipolar symptoms. Given that many untreated patients with bipolar disorder have low impulse control and a tendency to engage in risky behavior, the possibility for head injury becomes particularly pertinent.

For an individual first seen with symptoms, the physician should conduct a physical and neurological assessment, including blood work and thyroid function, to assess the possibility of these physiological disorders.

Physicians should assess these baseline chemistries prior to starting medications. While brain tumors and arterial-venous malformations are rare causes of bipolar disorder symptoms, physicians should consider a brain scan for those patients for whom one has never been conducted.

Conducting the Clinical Interview

A thorough clinical interview is an invaluable part of the assessment process. The interview provides a framework for understanding results of other assessment tools, such as questionnaires, as well as an opportunity to develop rapport and observe the patient's behavior, *affect*, and reactions to life events.

While clinical interviews can vary in the amount of structure provided, most will include some questions related to the patient's strengths, goals, nature and history of the problem, diagnosis, and relevant personal and family history. Although not comprehensive, the clinical areas covered in the checklist in figure 2.3 (on the next page) can help with diagnosis and treatment planning.

Research has also shown that the abuse of some drugs, including cocaine and steroids, can produce bipolar-like symptoms.

affect — the conscious subjective aspect of an emotion considered apart from bodily changes

Figure 2.3 Clinical Interview Checklist

	Assessment Topics	Rationale
Problem History	• Description of symptoms, including extent to which they disrupt/disturb ability to function • Initial onset of symptoms • Intensity and duration of symptoms consistent with hypomania, mania, and depression • Changes in frequency or character of symptoms over time • Antecedents/consequences of symptoms • History of prior treatment/attempts to resolve symptoms	To gain insight into the course of illness for the individual, increase motivation for treatment, and target new treatment approaches in which the patient may be more compliant
Personal/Developmental Background	• Infancy – developmental milestones, early medical history • Family atmosphere, characterization of family of origin, relationships • School adjustment and performance • Medical history • Family history of psychiatric illness and treatment response, including any history of suicide	To help identify family history of any mood or other psychiatric disorders, distinguish medical factors that may be important, identify the degree to which symptoms may have impacted academic performance, and target educational needs to enable the patient to become an informed participant in their treatment
Relationships	• Interpersonal relationships over time • Relationship/marriage history • Current social supports • Description of current living situation, relationships	To help assess the type and degree of social support available to the individual as well as the extent to which symptoms may have impaired the ability to engage in fulfilling and successful personal relationships
Financial/Occupational Background	• Work history • Current work status, performance, and satisfaction • Career goals • Economic stability	To help assess the difference between work reality, function, and goals. Those living with economic instability have additional pressures that may impact response to treatment; this pressure may add to depressive symptoms or foster choices inconsistent with treatment, like working several jobs around the clock.
Miscellaneous/ Other	• Fears, concerns, worries • Self-concept • Social/recreational activities/outlets • History of legal problems • Drug and/or alcohol use	To learn important goals/concerns of the patient. Additionally, information about history may confirm past symptom severity (e.g., accumulating huge financial debt and lawsuits due to gambling while manic). Current use of drugs and/or alcohol can negatively impact the course of the disorder and treatment response.

Appendix B offers information on specific tools, including suicide assessment measures.

Using Structured Symptom Evaluation Tools

Symptom evaluation tools clarify diagnoses and include structured clinical interviews, clinician-administered observational rating scales, self-ratings, and general assessments of psychiatric symptoms.

Structured Clinical Interviews

Highly structured diagnostic interviews were developed to reduce the emphasis on clinician judgment present in open-ended interviews. These interviews may require specialized training to administer correctly and can be time consuming. However, they have the benefit of objective criteria for diagnostic decisions. Some examples are:[36-38]

- ▶ The Schedule for Affective Disorders and Schizophrenia (SADS)
- ▶ Diagnostic Interview Schedule (DIS)
- ▶ The Structured Clinical Interview for the DSM-IV (SCID)

Clinician-Administered Observational Rating Scales

Many assessment tools combine structured to semi-structured interviews with behavioral observations. A trained interviewer conducts the face-to-face interviews and rates discrete symptom domains. These instruments incorporate information obtained through behavioral observations, and in some cases, collateral information, such as reports from family members or other clinicians. There are many published scales to measure symptoms of hypomania and mania. Some of the most commonly used scales include:[39, 40]

- ▶ Young Mania Rating Scale (YMRS)
- ▶ Clinician Administered Rating Scale for Mania – (CARS-M)

While there are many published scales to measure symptoms of **depression**, some of the most commonly used scales include:[41-47]

- ▶ Inventory of Depressive Symptomatology – Clinician-Rated (IDS-C)
- ▶ Hamilton Rating Scale for Depression (HAM-D) and the structured interview companion to the instrument
- ▶ Montgomery-Äsberg Depression Rating Scale (MADRS)

Self-Ratings

Patients can report their own symptoms using self-report, pencil-and-paper symptom inventories. These tools are appropriate for those patients who have *insight* and awareness of small but significant changes in mood that may precipitate a mood episode. Self ratings are inappropriate for patients who:

insight — understanding or awareness of one's mental or emotional condition

▶ Are not forthcoming with information

▶ Have limited insight into their symptoms and illness

▶ Are severely ill and possibly unable to accurately complete these self-administered reports

▶ Have problems with extensive reading

Self-report instruments developed specifically for comprehensive reporting of bipolar disorder symptoms are:[48-52]

▶ The Life Chart Method

▶ The Internal State Scale (ISS)

See appendix C for a sample log from the Life Chart.

Additionally, the Mood Disorder Questionnaire (MDQ) is a brief, self-report **diagnostic** instrument that screens for bipolar disorder.[53] A new version of the MDQ, MDQ-Expanded, screens for current symptoms of mania, depression, and alcohol abuse.[54]

Other self-report tools measure either hypomania/mania or depression independently. These tools include:[41, 55-58]

▶ The Altman Mania Rating Scale (AMRS)

▶ The Inventory for Depressive Symptoms – Self Report (IDS-SR)

▶ The Beck Depression Inventory (BDI-2)

Appendix B offers information on specific tools, including suicide assessment measures.

General Psychiatric Symptom Assessment Tools

A trained clinician might also choose to use a general measure of psychiatric symptoms and/or personality function to assist in the diagnostic process. These tools can help pinpoint other psychiatric symptoms that can co-occur with symptoms of mania and depression. Alternatively, there are many high-quality, published interviews and self-report instruments that assess symptoms of psychosis, anxiety, anger, somatization, and other psychiatric symptoms that may be helpful to include in individual assessments as needed.

Appendix B offers information on specific tools, including suicide assessment measures.

While the measures listed below are not specific to symptoms of bipolar disorder, they can be helpful in differentiating presenting symptoms from those consistent with other disorders:[59-62]

- ▶ The Brief Psychiatric Rating Scale (BPRS)
- ▶ The Minnesota Multiphasic Personality Inventory – 2nd Edition (MMPI)
- ▶ The Millon Clinical Multiaxial Inventory (MCMI)

Assessing Suicide Risk

Bipolar disorder is accompanied by a high risk for self-injury and suicide when untreated or when patients experience limited response to treatment.[21, 22] Those with comorbid alcohol or substance abuse or dependence are at greater risk for suicide, as are those who have made previous suicide attempts. Assessment of suicide risk is a complex and multidimensional task, and should be an ongoing aspect of interactions between care providers and the patient.

In addition to assessing general domains, the clinician must consider the context in which these thoughts are occurring. The severity of depression, anger, impulsivity, use of drugs or alcohol, events in the person's life, and other variables must all be considered when evaluating the risk for suicide.

There are multiple assessment tools designed to assist clinicians in assessing suicide risk. Most of these include some assessment of these general domains:

- ▶ The wish to live or die
- ▶ Experience of impulses related to suicide as well as control over these impulses
- ▶ Duration and frequency of suicidal ideation (thoughts)
- ▶ Specificity of ideas or plans for suicide
- ▶ Access to lethal means
- ▶ Deterrents to suicide (e.g., support from family members, religious beliefs)
- ▶ Any active preparation for suicide (e.g., writing letters to loved ones, giving away dear possessions)

The following describes some assessment tools that may be helpful in routine clinical assessment of suicide risk.

- ▶ **Beck Scale for Suicide Ideation (BSS; self-administered version)** — The BSS is a 21-item, self-report scale that is completed independently by the patient. Higher scores indicate increasing suicidal ideation and risk. As this scale takes about five to 10 minutes to complete, it can be useful as part of a package of assessment tools completed prior to routine visits. However, it should not substitute for face-to-face assessment of recent suicidal thoughts or plans.

▶ **Scale for Suicide Ideation (SSI; clinician-administered version)** — The SSI is administered in an approximately 10-minute interview with a clinician and can assess either current ideation or worst ideation ever experienced. It includes the same 21 items contained on the self-report version, the Beck Scale for Suicide Ideation, described above. The SSI provides a reliable, valid, and rapid method of systematically estimating suicidal ideation.

▶ **Suicide Intent Scale (SIS)** — The SIS is designed to measure the intensity of the attempter's wish to die at the time of the attempt and is typically administered to an individual after a suicide attempt. This scale has primarily been used in research settings, although the intensity of the person's wish to die is viewed as an important risk factor for future suicide attempts. The SIS includes 20 items, and it is administered by a trained clinician in a brief interview.

Collected retrospectively, the SSI results are subject to some bias, depending on the length of elapsed time or other factors that may obscure memory for the event.

▶ **Beck Hopelessness Scale (BHS)** — The BHS is a 20-item, true-false scale that can be completed independently by the patient in five to 10 minutes. Hopelessness correlates with the overall severity of depression and may be more related to risk for suicide than other symptoms of depression. Higher scores on the BHS, suggesting greater hopelessness, are associated with eventual suicide attempt or completion.[63, 64] Hopelessness is not related to immediate risk, but rather, risk over time. Fortunately, scores on the BHS decrease with successful treatment for depression.[63]

Hopelessness is an indirect measure of suicidality, as those with greater pessimism about the future may be at greater risk for suicide.

What Differentiates Bipolar Disorder from Other Disorders?

Bipolar disorder is a psychiatric illness very likely to co-exist with other psychiatric conditions, implying for many with these coexisting conditions that resolving bipolar disorder symptoms may be slower, and there may be a need for other treatments to directly address symptoms of the comorbid condition(s). Given the susceptibility of patients with bipolar disorder to become manic (BD-I) or hypomanic (BD-II) with use of certain medications, a careful balancing and monitoring of medications is often required. For example, if an antidepressant or stimulant medication is added to improve energy and goal-directed behavior, a patient with BD-I must be on adequate anti-manic treatment to avoid a risk of new manic symptoms.

When diagnosing bipolar disorder, the clinician must rule out the possibility that the individual's symptoms are related to:

- ▶ Major Depressive Disorder
- ▶ Substance-Induced Mood Disorder
- ▶ Mood Disorder due to a General Medical Condition
- ▶ Attention Deficit Hyperactivity Disorder
- ▶ Psychotic Disorders

Many patients request help during depressive episodes, and if not queried specifically, clinicians may miss the history of hypomania or mania.

Major Depressive Disorder — The most challenging differential diagnosis for clinicians is distinguishing bipolar disorder from unipolar depression, particularly in patients who experience hypomania and not mania (BD-II). Patients may not recognize or correctly label periods of hypomania, particularly mixed hypomania. Thorough questioning of the individual and/or family, or other collateral informants, regarding lifetime occurrence of one or more episodes of hypomania or mania will resolve this issue. If there is a history of at least one manic episode, the patient meets criteria for bipolar I disorder. If there is a history of hypomania, criteria for BD-II are met.

When substance-induced mood disorder is suspected, appropriate laboratory tests and screenings should be performed to determine the exact etiology of mood symptoms.

Substance-Induced Mood Disorder — A substance-induced mood disorder is a significant mood disturbance caused by the use of a substance (e.g., a drug of abuse, alcohol, a medication, or exposure to a toxin). Use or withdrawal from substances, such as cocaine, amphetamines, or alcohol, may produce symptoms similar to mania and/or depression, and these episodes should be described as a substance-induced mood disorder.

The clinician should specifically ask the patient about the onset of symptoms and the use of substances. For example, intoxication from cocaine may mimic a manic episode, and would be described as a cocaine-induced mood disorder, with manic features, according to DSM-IV (TR) criteria. If symptoms do not remit after withdrawal of the substance and an appropriate time interval, the diagnosis of a bipolar disorder should be reconsidered.

Physiological conditions that can produce bipolar-like symptoms:

- ▶ *Embolic stroke*
- ▶ *A hyperthyroid or a hypothyroid condition*
- ▶ *Temporal lobe epilepsy*
- ▶ *Neoplastic or cancer syndromes*
- ▶ *Abuse of some drugs, including cocaine and steroids*
- ▶ *Head injuries*

Mood Disorder Due to a General Medical Condition — This diagnosis is reserved for mood symptoms judged to be a direct physiological consequence of a specific general medical condition. Certain medical conditions (e.g., brain tumor, Cushing's syndrome, or hypothyroidism) can mimic symptoms of either mania or depression. This determination can be made by a thorough medical history, laboratory findings, or physical examination.

Generally, if a patient is non-responsive to treatments for bipolar disorder, the clinician should reconsider the diagnosis and perform further diagnostic tests to rule out other causes or contributing medical factors.

Attention Deficit Hyperactivity Disorder (ADHD) — ADHD must be differentiated from hypomania or mania, as they share the characteristics of impulsivity, poor judgment, and excessive activity. This differentiation is best accomplished by obtaining a thorough developmental history. Consider ADHD if:

> ► Symptoms of inattention, hyperactivity, or impulsivity consistently occurred prior to the age of seven.

> ► Early school history is characterized by persistent teacher complaints of such behaviors and disruption in learning.

ADHD is also characterized by a chronic course, while bipolar symptoms tend to be more **episodic**. Additionally, those with bipolar disorder have specific mood symptoms, such as sustained episodes of significant depression, which may or may not be present in those with ADHD.

Unlike other mood or psychotic disorders, ADHD can be diagnosed as a comorbid condition in those with bipolar disorder.

Psychotic Disorders — Psychotic disorders and BD-I can share a number of symptoms, including grandiose and persecutory delusions, irritability, withdrawal, and agitation. This overlap is most pronounced early in the course of all disorders, before full symptoms of the disorder are present. However, diagnosis of all the psychotic disorders requires the presence of psychotic symptoms in the absence of prominent mood symptoms. In bipolar disorder, psychotic symptoms will occur with mood symptoms during the course of either depressive or manic episodes. Other areas that may help differentiate diagnoses are the type of accompanying symptoms, previous course, and family psychiatric history.

Psychotic disorders include: schizoaffective disorder, schizophrenia, schizophreniform disorder, delusional disorder, and psychotic disorder not otherwise specified.

Anxiety Disorders — The prominent clinical presentation in multiple anxiety disorders is chronic and debilitating anxiety, versus fluctuating mood episodes on the bipolar spectrum.

Persons with anxiety disorders present as chronically worried or fearful, and have corresponding reductions in their ability to function as a result of those fears.

It is possible to have a diagnosis of both bipolar disorder and an anxiety disorder. Therefore, the critical issue is not necessarily in differentiating bipolar symptoms from anxiety, but rather, in determining whether coexisting anxiety symptoms may be present and require clinical attention as well.

Anxiety disorders include:
► Acute stress disorder
► Agoraphobia without history of panic disorder
► Anxiety disorder due to general medical condition
► Generalized anxiety disorder
► Obsessive-compulsive disorder
► Panic disorder with agoraphobia
► Panic disorder without agoraphobia
► Post-traumatic stress disorder
► Specific phobia
► Social phobia
► Substance-induced anxiety disorder
► Anxiety disorder NOS

How Does Bipolar Disorder Present in Children and Adolescents?

Symptoms of bipolar disorder may be difficult to recognize in children and adolescents, as they can be mistaken for age-appropriate emotions and behaviors. Symptoms of mania and depression may appear in a variety of behaviors. **When manic**, children and adolescents, in contrast to adults, are more likely to be irritable and prone to destructive outbursts than to be elated or euphoric. **When depressed**, there may be complaints of headaches, stomach aches, tiredness, poor school performance, poor communication, and extreme sensitivity to rejection or failure.

According to the American Academy of Child and Adolescent Psychiatry, up to one-third of the 3.4 million children and adolescents with depression in the U.S. may actually be experiencing the early onset of bipolar disorder.

Treating bipolar disorder in children relies on experience in treating adults with the illness, since very few studies have been done of the effectiveness and safety of the medications currently used for adults when given to children and adolescents. Pediatric treatment guidelines for bipolar disorder have recently been generated based on available evidence and expert consensus.[65]

Key Concepts for Chapter Two:

1. Thorough assessment for the historical presence of hypomanic or manic symptoms is essential in differentiating bipolar disorder from unipolar depression.

2. Bipolar disorder is characterized by episodes of depression, hypomania, and/or mania, or for mixed episodes.

3. Individuals with untreated bipolar disorder, or those unresponsive to treatment, are at increased risk for suicide.

4. In the DSM-IV (TR), recognized diagnoses for bipolar spectrum disorders include BD-I, BD-II, BD-NOS, and cyclothymic disorder.

5. Rapid cycling is specified when the person experiences four or more episodes in a year. These patients may be less responsive to treatment.

6. There are many options and approaches to assessing of bipolar disorder, including medical evaluation, clinical interview, and structured symptom assessments.

7. Other disorders can cause "bipolar-like" symptoms. It is important to differentiate bipolar disorder from major depressive disorder, substance-induced mood disorder, mood disorder due to a medical condition, and ADHD as well as psychotic and anxiety disorders.

Chapter 3:
Biological Treatment of Bipolar Disorder

This chapter answers the following:

- ▶ **What is the Role of Genetics in Bipolar Disorder?** — This section reviews research on the genetic inheritance of bipolar disorder.

- ▶ **How does Brain Anatomy and Physiology differ for Patients with Bipolar Disorder?** — This section covers how neuroimaging studies have helped define the areas of the brain involved in bipolar disorder.

- ▶ **What Medications are used to Treat Mania/Hypomania in Patients with Bipolar Disorder?** — This section covers medications for mania and hypomania, including treatment strategies and efficacy as well as using combination medications.

- ▶ **What Medications are used to Treat Depression in Patients with Bipolar Disorder?** — This section covers medications for depression, including treatment strategies and efficacy.

- ▶ **What Strategies are Recommended for Maintenance Treatment?** — This section provides recently published recommendations and efficacy information on maintenance treatment for patients with bipolar disorder.

- ▶ **How can Medication Treatment of Side Effects be Managed?** — This section presents strategies for treating the side effects sometimes experienced with bipolar medication treatment.

- ▶ **How are Electroconvulsive Therapy (ECT) and Alternative Medicine Used to Treat Bipolar Disorder?** — This section discusses electroconvulsive therapy (ECT) and other non-medication biological approaches.

- ▶ **How Does Comorbidity Impact Medication Treatment for Bipolar Disorder?** — This section addresses the impact of comorbid disorders on medication treatment strategies.

IN recent decades, we've come to understand that bipolar disorder typically stems from instability and malfunction in brain activity, not from environmental causes. However, we continue to have a limited and rudimentary understanding of the exact mechanisms underlying the disorder. The field is advancing at a rapid rate as findings in brain research and the neurosciences expand.

During depression, the frontal cortex will show decreased activation; during mania, temporal lobe regions will show increased activation. Researchers believe that changes in activation can be correlated with blood flow and brain activity.

What is the Role of Genetics in Bipolar Disorder?

When seeing patients, it is very important to ask what other family members may have bipolar disorder, depression, or a history of substance abuse.

Based on recent research, bipolar disorder is now recognized as an inherited illness where a number of genes interact to make an individual more vulnerable to develop the disorder.[66.]

Several respected European adoption studies have found that the possibility of developing bipolar disorder to be higher for children who had a birth parent diagnosed with bipolar disorder, whether or not the child was raised with that individual.[67, 68] In fact, the frequency of bipolar disorder is significantly higher in parents and children of those with bipolar disorder. In addition, twin studies indicate a much higher risk for identical twins (50 percent) than for fraternal twins (about 15–20 percent).[2]

When one parent has bipolar disorder, the risk to each child can be 15–20 percent. When both parents have bipolar disorder, the risk increases to 50–75 percent.

Among family members with bipolar disorder, the risk for other psychiatric illnesses is significantly elevated as well. For any given individual with bipolar disorder, the likelihood of family members having depression is significant, at least as much as bipolar disorder itself. The risk for other, co-existing psychiatric illnesses is also high, including substance abuse and anxiety disorders. Members of families in which more than one person has bipolar disorder or depression can experience both earlier onset and a more severe course of bipolar disorder.[5, 15]

Stress management is an important component for any patient with bipolar disorder. An individual with the illness is vulnerable to developing clinical symptoms of bipolar disorder when stressed. For example, sleep deprivation or a significant psychosocial stress could predispose someone currently stable to experience a new episode. Although currently unproven by research, some theorists also suggest that patients may carry the genetic predisposi-

From the Patient's Perspective

The doctor says there is a connection between all my energy right now and the way I was feeling last winter, and that I have something called, "bipolar disorder." Now, I'm supposed to take "mood stabilizing" medication. I didn't think that these problems were that bad, and I am a little surprised that she thinks I need medicine. However, I've been on it for a few weeks now, and I do feel better. I am getting better sleep, and feel more in control of myself. Hopefully, it will prevent me from getting depressed again too. I am going to miss that extra energy, but she says that bipolar disorder is a biological illness, and I have to take it seriously and do this treatment so it won't get worse.

tion to bipolar disorder, but not develop symptoms unless exposed to significant stress, especially during developmental periods. For example, extensive use of illegal substances or early physical or sexual trauma could trigger this stress-vulnerability.

How does Brain Anatomy and Physiology differ for Patients with Bipolar Disorder?

This section addresses specific brain areas involved in the disorder as well as relevant biochemical and physiological factors and secondary messenger systems within nerve cells.

Specific Brain Areas Involved in Bipolar Disorder

Brain areas involved when people are depressed and manic include the frontal lobe (where the brain performs many of its *executive* and organizational functions) and temporal lobes (involved in regulating emotions). For years, theorists implicated the *temporal lobe,* which includes the *hippocampus* and the *amygdala*, in the development of affective instability, including depression, bipolar disorder, and aggression. For example, those with epilepsy syndromes localized to the temporal lobe (specifically, the hippocampus) develop many bipolar-like symptoms, including unstable moods and *paranormal phenomena*. Figure 3.1 illustrates the specific brain areas impacted by bipolar disorder.

Figure 3.1   Brain Areas Impacted by Bipolar Disorder

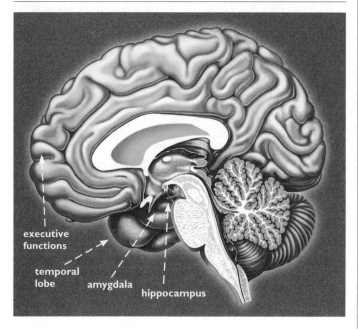

executive functions — those functions of the brain carried out by the prefrontal and frontal cortex: managing stimuli, marshalling appropriate responses, and modulating impulses, which are all disrupted in the manic state

temporal lobe — a large lobe of each cerebral hemisphere that is in front of the occipital lobe and is believed to be involved in memory, mood regulation, and impulsivity

hippocampus — an important part of the limbic system involved in working memory and other functions

amygdala — one of the basal ganglia that is part of the limbic system and believed to be involved in impulsivity and other functions

paranormal phenomena — altered perceptions experienced by the patient but not those around them, [e.g., hearing voices (auditory hallucinations), smelling burning rubber (olfactory hallucinations), etc.] as well as déjà vu, the sense of having already experienced what is now happening

With current neuroimaging technology — PET and *SPECT imaging* — we can now:

- ▶ Identify some brain areas involved in the disorder
- ▶ Establish that the brain is physiologically different, depending on the mood state the person is experiencing
- ▶ Assess differences in patients' brains when they experience depression versus mania versus euthymia (see figure 3.2 below for an example)
- ▶ Demonstrate how brain function normalizes after medication treatment, indicating that medications effectively return brain activity to more balanced function

Figure 3.2   Brain Function by SPECT Imaging Scan

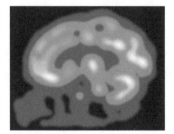   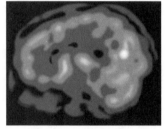

Mania   No Clinical Evidence of Mania

We cannot, at present, use neuroimaging technologies to diagnose a specific illness or to predict the most effective treatment approach.

Biochemical and Physiological Factors Related to Bipolar Disorder

neurotransmitter — a chemical in the brain that transmits information between the nerve cells

major neurochemical receptor groups — neurotransmitter substances believed important in normal and abnormal brain functioning

dopamine — a neurotransmitter in the central nervous system that affects the synthesis of epinephrine

serotonin — a neurotransmitter from the indoleamine group that affects central nervous system functioning

atypical antipsychotics — the class of antipsychotic medications with less extrapyramidal side-effects

Much of the biochemical theory about bipolar disorder stems from our understanding of drug mechanisms, expanding as novel medications have been found effective in the treatment of this illness. Nineteenth century thinking was that mental illnesses and bipolar disorder were due to the deposit of salt on the brain tissue itself. As a result, by the mid-1800s, lithium bromide was recommended by physicians to treat mania and melancholia as both an acute and prophylactic treatment. As our understanding of the physiologic bases of brain activity became increasingly sophisticated, this potentially effective treatment was lost until the 1950s.[69] While earlier schools of thought debated what caused bipolar disorder — whether the *neurotransmitter*, norepinephrine, regulated moods or that *dopamine* was related to psychoses — researchers now understand that interactions producing both abnormal brain states and relative stability are much more complex than originally thought. For example, in evaluating how *atypical antipsychotics* impact the brain's *major neurochemical receptor group,* debate continues as to whether more *serotonin* versus less serotonin, more dopamine versus less dopamine (or the combination of the two) are the critical components of mood stabilization.

Secondary Messenger Systems

Historically, psychiatric research focused on receptor activity (i.e., the activity at the cell surface). Now, many studies are ongoing to better understand the specific mechanisms inside the neuronal cell associated with both symptoms of bipolar disorder and how medications to treat bipolar disorder act on the brain. Studies focusing on these mechanisms in patients treated with lithium and other compounds (especially anticonvulsant medications) suggest a disruption (e.g., too much or too little of a second messenger molecule) and that lithium corrects this imbalance, leading to mood stabilization.

This focus on second messengers has also led to an awareness of a *neuroprotective effect* of many mood stabilization medications. Lithium and many of the anticonvulsants appear to have a protective effect in animal models where there is a decreased loss of already existing cells and evidence showing an increased likelihood of new neurogenesis.[70]

New areas of research are also focusing on brain effects of:

▶ **Neuropeptides** — Brain chemicals or medications that either decrease cell death and/or increase neurogenesis.

▶ **Cotransmitters** — Two molecules released from the same synapse that act on an adjacent neuron, both of which are physiologically active.

▶ **Hormone receptors** (e.g., steroid receptors) — A group of molecules that have diverse function throughout the brain and the body (e.g., estrogen).

▶ **Neurotrophins** — A class of molecules whose effects occur through specific cell membrane receptors that trigger changes in the second messenger system(s). These effects range from increased cell survival to increased new cell growth.

As a result, we can expect important new findings in the next 10 years on fundamental brain processes and underlying mechanisms of major psychiatric illnesses.

Although there is no cure for bipolar disorder, in most cases it can be treated and controlled with medication. Treatment options have increased significantly over the past 20 years beyond lithium, which was the primary treatment option for bipolar disorder until the 1980s. While lithium is helpful for both depressive and hypomanic/manic symptoms, other medications are also effective for treating mood states. For example, recent discoveries demonstrate that anticonvulsant medications may be used for treating mood instability, (e.g., divalproex and carbamazepine). Additionally, current research focuses on the extent to which bipolar disorder symptoms may be successfully

neuroprotective effect — the function of a brain chemical or medication to either decrease cell death and/or increase the birth of new brain cells (i.e., neurogenesis)

Research in recent years has turned to the next level of brain function — secondary messenger systems — neurochemical systems used to carry and communicate activity from a cell's surface throughout the cell body and into the areas that determine the cell's genetic products.

Our increasing knowledge and understanding of brain function leads to better and more-specific drug development. Observing responses to specific medications likewise informs us regarding brain function and processes.

Only a few medications have FDA approval for treatment of specific episodes in bipolar disorder. Others may have evidence to support their use, but are not yet through the approval process. Use of non-FDA-approved medications (termed, "off-label") for treating bipolar disorder is frequent.

It is important to note that all medication use *must balance benefits and risks to particular patients. For example, the FDA recently issued a public health advisory, warning of increased mortality among elderly patients receiving atypical antipsychotics for treatment of dementia-related behavioral disorders.*

For full information about medications, clinicians should carefully review package inserts for individual medications or access the **Physicians Desk Reference** *(PDR).*

treated with the new-generation, atypical antipsychotic medications (e.g., aripiprazole, olanzapine, quetiapine, risperidone, or ziprasidone). While individuals diagnosed with bipolar disorder require lifetime monitoring and treatment, many can achieve and maintain stable moods for long periods.

Medication recommendations are generally developed from research on patients with bipolar I disorder (BD-I). Conservative estimates suggest there may be at least as many bipolar II disorder (BD-II) and bipolar disorder – not otherwise specified (BD-NOS) patients as BD-I patients, supporting the need for research to help delineate the most appropriate treatment. It is possible that patients diagnosed with BD-II or BD-NOS will benefit equally from these treatments, but little research has been done to isolate or specify treatments for these groups.

As many as 50 percent of patients with BD-I experience psychotic symptoms when in a manic or mixed state. However, these symptoms are viewed as part of the illness, and in most cases, respond to mania treatment. Therefore, this text does not specifically address treating psychotic symptoms.

What Medications are used to Treat Mania/Hypomania in Patients with Bipolar Disorder?

Medications for treating mania/hypomania symptoms include lithium, anticonvulsants, and atypical antipsychotic drugs as well as combination medications. While they all act on the brain to decrease manic, mixed, or hypomanic symptoms (e.g., an antimanic effect), they each have different mechanisms of action. Complicated sets of checks and balances exist within cells, and it is likely that medications fundamentally work by decreasing or modifying cell activity, leading to cellular balance that minimizes altered behavior and clinical syndromes. For example, valproate (VPA) and carbamazepine (CBZ) are both anticonvulsants that decrease excessive excitability and enhance the brain's inhibitory functions responsible for providing checks and balances in brain cell activity. However, valproate also acts on calcium ionic channels and may impact secondary messenger systems differently than CBZ.

Figure 3.3 (on pages 32 and 33) summarizes recommended doses and more common side effects for each of the mania/hypomania treatments discussed in this section. This information has been compiled from the **Physicians Desk Reference** and the TMAP physician manual.[71, 72] These medications are effective for acute mania and mixed states, returning brain function to more normalized states. They have been researched in *evidence-based studies* of patients with bipolar I disorder. As symptoms decrease, sleep increases, irritability decreases, moods are more even, and the patient is able to concentrate and gradually resume usual activities. Untreated mania was observed to last six to 10 weeks prior to the use of medications. Medication treatment minimizes symptoms in days, though full symptom resolution often requires three to four weeks.

Lithium — In 1970, lithium became the first drug to receive U.S. Food and Drug Administration (FDA) approval for the treatment of manic episodes in bipolar disorder. Lithium (Li) also has an FDA indication for maintenance treatment for preventing new episodes.

Anticonvulsants — A number of research results indicate that certain anticonvulsant medications are helpful for treating mania and/or mixed states, especially:

- ▶ Divalproex (FDA-approved treatment for mania)
- ▶ Carbamazepine - extended release (FDA-approved treatment for mania and mixed episodes)
- ▶ Lamotrigine (FDA approved as a *maintenance treatment* for prevention of new bipolar mood episodes)

Atypical Antipsychotic Medications — This group of medications represents a significant breakthrough for patients with schizophrenia and bipolar disorder. Unlike the "typical" or older antipsychotics, these medications (as a group) cause fewer, less severe, or no movement disorder side effects, such as dystonia, akathisia, and others.

The atypical antipsychotic medications, which have anti-manic properties, include:

- ▶ Aripiprazole (FDA-approved treatment for acute mania and mixed episodes)
- ▶ Clozapine (FDA-approved treatment for schizophrenia; a good treatment option for patients who have failed other treatments, are compliant with the required monitoring, and who are free of contraindicated medical conditions)
- ▶ Olanzapine [FDA-approved treatment for acute mania and mixed episodes as well as for both maintenance and, in combination with fluoxetine (an SSRI), treatment of acute bipolar depression]
- ▶ Risperidone (FDA-approved treatment for acute mania and mixed episodes)
- ▶ Quetiapine (FDA-approved treatment for acute mania)
- ▶ Ziprasidone (FDA-approved treatment for acute mania and mixed episodes)

---

evidence-based studies — medication information gained through placebo-controlled, double-blind studies (where neither the patient nor physician know who receives the "active" pill with medication versus the "sugar" pill)

Taking frequent blood levels helps ensure therapeutic dosing when utilizing many anticonvulsants.

Oxcarbazepine *(structurally similar to carbamazepine) has been studied in open, uncontrolled trials; however, there is no current FDA indication for bipolar disorder.*

maintenance treatment — an ongoing treatment believed to prevent or minimize the development of new episodes of mania, depression, or mixed states

Lamotrigine is not indicated for treatment of acute mania or mixed episodes. For more detailed information on lamotrigine for treating bipolar depression, see pages 40, 41, and 44.

Figure 3.3   Medication Dosages and Common Side Effects for Treating Acute Phase of Mania/Hypomania in Patients with Bipolar Disorder*

Type/Class: Medication*	Usual Target Dose	Usual Maximum Recommended Dose (level)	Recommended Administration Schedule	Common Side Effects**
Lithium**	0.6–1.0 mEq/L	1.2 mEq/L	2 times daily or at bedtime	Tremor, drowsiness, nausea/vomiting, increased urine output, muscle weakness, thirst, dry mouth, cognitive impairment
Anticonvulsants:				
Valproate** (divalproex is the FDA-approved formulation for bipolar disorder)	80 ug/mL	125 ug/mL	2 times daily or at bedtime	Nausea/vomiting, increased appetite with weight gain, sedation, hair loss, reversible increases in liver function tests, reversible thrombocytopenia, rarely pancreatitis
Carbamazepine** (carbamazepine-ERC*** is the FDA-approved formulation for bipolar disorder)	4–12 ug/mL 400–1600 mg/day	12 ug/mL 1600 mg/day	2 times daily	Dizziness, drowsiness, blurred vision, fatigue, nausea, vomiting, ataxia
Oxcarbazepine	600–2400 mg/day	2400 mg/day	2 times daily or at bedtime	Dizziness, below-normal sodium range in the blood, rapid involuntary eyeball movements, headache, sedation, impaired speech, double vision

*This review of medications is intended to provide information on commonly used medications and upcoming changes, but not to be comprehensive. Additionally, this information is not intended to provide prescription information, and a physician or appropriate individual should be consulted prior to making medication changes. For full information about medications, physicians should carefully review package inserts for individual medications or access the *Physicians Desk Reference.*

Side effects may be less with slow-absorbing forms of medications. Lithium, valproate, and carbamazepine are also available in slow-absorption (or extended-release) formulations.

***Therapeutic blood levels are not required for carbamazepine ERC.

Figure 3.3 continued

Type/Class: Medication*	Usual Target Dose**	Usual Maximum Recommended Dose (level)	Recommended Administration Schedule	Common Side Effects***
Atypical Antipsychotics (AAPs):				
Aripiprazole	15–30 mg/day	30 mg/day	once daily	Sedation, Parkinson-like symptoms,**** internal feeling of restlessness or agitation (akathisia)
Clozapine	100–300 mg/day	900 mg/day	at bedtime	Sedation, weight gain,*** dry mouth, constipation, and potential mental confusion, abrupt drop in blood pressure when suddenly changing from lying to sitting or sitting to standing, rapid heart rate, excessive salivation, constipation, nausea, and vomiting
Olanzapine	10–15 mg/day	20 mg/day	2 times daily or at bedtime	Sedation, weight gain, dry mouth, constipation, and potential mental confusion, mild Parkinson-like symptoms,**** and slowed movements
Quetiapine	500–600 mg/day	800 mg/day	2 times daily or at bedtime	Sedation, orthostatic hypotension, weight gain; potential thyroid inhibition
Risperidone	2–4 mg/day	6 mg/day	2 times daily or at bedtime	Sedation, Parkinson-like symptoms,**** weight gain, hypotension, sexual dysfunction; elevated prolactin
Ziprasidone	120–160 mg/day	160 mg/day	2 times daily	Sedation, nausea and vomiting, constipation, Parkinson-like symptoms,**** dizziness

   * This review of medications is intended to provide information on commonly used medications and upcoming changes, but not to be comprehensive. Additionally, this information is not intended to provide prescription information and a physician or appropriate individual should be consulted prior to making medication changes.

  **Doses used for maintenance treatment may be lower.

***General notes on AAP side effects:
    (1) Severity of weight gain generally rated as: Clozapine = olanzapine > quetiapine = risperidone > aripiprazole = ziprasidone.
    (2) Relative risks of newer antipsychotics for causing tardive dyskinesia are still being studied.

****These symptoms include flat facial expression, stiff muscles, and slowed movements.

An exciting new development is that, as well as decreasing manic and mixed symptoms, these medications may also decrease depressive symptoms when given to a patient with bipolar disorder who is acutely depressed. Positive, placebo-controlled data are available supporting this for olanzapine and quetiapine, and open data support this for other members of this medication class (see the efficacy discussion on page 37).

Current research for atypical antipsychotic agents focuses on developing usage guidelines, linking specific agents with differing clinical symptom patterns, and addressing long-term safety and tolerance issues. Each of the medications listed in the charts above has a somewhat different impact on brain receptors. Thus, while one medication may be less effective in an individual, another medication from this class may be more effective due to differences in:

> ► How the medication changes activity of brain neurons or effects different brain receptors

> ► What side effects different patients experience

Using Treatment Algorithms and Guidelines for Bipolar Patients

algorithms — an organized, often specific set of recommendations that are evidence-based, often informed by expert consensus opinion when there are inadequate studies to inform treatment decisions

Using medication *algorithms* and guidelines allows the clinician to use treatment approaches based on new data and expert experience treating particular patient groups. Evidence-based algorithms for the treatment of bipolar disorder are available to guide clinical decision-making and treatment. One example, the Texas Implementation of Medication Algorithms (TIMA) program, develops evidence-based medication guidelines. TIMA's most recent guideline for treating BD-I hypomanic/manic episodes is presented in figure 3.4 on page 35 and illustrates one type of algorithm presentation.[73]

TIMA's recent algorithms reflect the consensus panel decisions made in May 2004, when a diverse group of academic psychiatrists and clinical psychopharmacology specialists met to review the newest available evidence for selecting treatments for bipolar disorder. Other members of the panel were Texas Department of State Health Services administrators as well as community mental health physicians, advocates, and consumers.

Other recently published guidelines for the treatment of bipolar disorder include the American Psychiatric Association Guidelines, Veterans Administration Guideline, and the Expert Consensus Guideline.[74-76]

When available, the panel based its decisions on evidence from well-controlled studies, employing a method similar to the one used by the Agency for Healthcare Research and Quality (AHRQ) to develop guidelines for treating depression.

The TIMA Treatment Algorithm for Hypomania/Mania

The algorithm for treating those currently hypomanic/manic differentiates between treatment for those experiencing euphoric versus mixed symptoms. Additionally, it recommends targeted adjunctive treatment for those with acute symptoms, using:

▶ Clonidine or sedatives for agitated/aggressive symptoms

▶ Hypnotics for insomnia

▶ Benzodiazepines or gabapentin for anxiety

> *For more information about the specific medications recommended in the TIMA 2005 treatment algorithms, refer to TIMA: Update to the Algorithms for Treatment of Bipolar I Disorder.[73]*

Figure 3.4   TIMA Algorithm for Treating Bipolar I Disorder, Currently Hypomanic/Manic (2005)

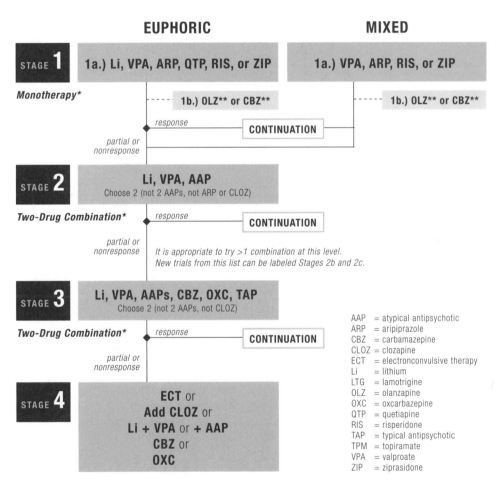

*Use targeted adjunctive treatment as necessary before moving to next stage:
  Agitation/Aggression — clonidine, sedatives
  Insomnia — hypnotics
  Anxiety — benzodiazepines, gabapentin

**Safety and other concerns led to placement of OLZ and CBZ as alternate 1st stage choices.

Effectiveness of Medications for Treating Mania/Hypomania Symptoms of Bipolar Disorder

Significant efficacy studies have been done for lithium, anticonvulsants, and atypical antipsychotics.

Lithium

Controlled studies have demonstrated that lithium is superior to placebo for treatment of acute mania when prescribed for one to three weeks at a therapeutic level.[77] However, much of this early research has been criticized for methodological problems, particularly the reliance on *crossover designs,* many of which abruptly discontinued lithium for those in the placebo group — an approach that may, in itself, cause or exacerbate bipolar symptoms.[78, 79] Other data suggest that patients with mixed mania, or dysphoric mania, respond better to anticonvulsants than lithium; therefore, lithium is not the first choice for patients with bipolar disorder with mixed presentations.[6]

crossover design — a type of clinical study where patients are randomized to one treatment arm, then at some point during the study will be "crossed over" to receive the other treatment option

Anticonvulsants

Research results indicate efficacy for divalproex (valproate), carbamazepine, and oxcarbazepine for treating bipolar hypomania/mania.

Divalproex (Valproate) — There are good, placebo-controlled data supporting this drug's efficacy as a single therapy for mania or mixed states.[80-81] Divalproex sodium, the enteric-coated form of valproate, was FDA approved for the treatment of acute mania in the early 1990s. In head-to-head studies with lithium, divalproex was more effective to decrease symptoms of mixed states.[6]

According to recently published research, women may be at risk of developing polycystic ovarian syndrome and hyperandrogenism soon after beginning valproate treatment.[82, 83] However, these studies found the risk to be lower than indicated in earlier, smaller studies.[84]

Carbamazepine — Similar to divalproex, this medication may be particularly helpful when depressive symptoms are present during mania.[2] Recent placebo-controlled studies in acute mania with the slow-absorbing form of carbamazepine support good effectiveness and tolerability for acute manic or mixed symptoms in bipolar disorder and led to FDA approval.[85, 86]

For TIMA 2005, the consensus panel placed carbamazepine within a substage (stage 1b) due to concerns over drug interaction and tolerability.[73] These concerns can be addressed through careful management, such as monitoring blood levels and side effects; however, therapeutic blood levels are not required for carbamazepine ERC.

Oxcarbazepine — This drug is structurally similar to carbamazepine and has comparable effectiveness in studies of epilepsy and in preliminary work in patients with bipolar disorder. Oxcarbazepine also does not require blood-level monitoring.[87-88] However, patients must be monitored for the medication's potential to lower sodium levels.

TIMA 2005 recommends oxcarbazepine as a stage-three medication (due to the lack of controlled studies) to be given in combination with those recommended for stage two.[73]

Atypical Antipsychotics

Recent studies conducted under double-blind, placebo-controlled conditions have shown antimanic properties of aripiprazole, olanzapine, quetiapine, risperidone, and ziprasidone.

Aripiprazole — FDA approved for acute mania and maintenance treatment, this medication has proven efficacious for both manic and mixed episodes in two multicenter, randomized, double-blind, placebo-controlled studies.[89, 90]

Clozapine — This was the first atypical antipsychotic whose efficacy in the most ill patients with schizophrenia led to significant efforts to develop other medications in this class over the last 20 years. While there have been no placebo-controlled studies in bipolar disorder, one open, controlled, one-year study and open monotherapy in acute mania support efficacy.[91, 92] Importantly, like patients with schizophrenia, these studies and others were done with more severely ill, treatment-resistant (i.e., refractory to treatment) patients with bipolar disorder.

Clozapine is an antipsychotic that has a clearly defined role in the treatment of refractory bipolar disorder, both as monotherapy and in combination with other psychotropic medications.[91, 93, 94]

Olanzapine — The effectiveness of this medication for reducing manic symptoms has been demonstrated in placebo-controlled and double-blind trials.[95-97] This medication has received FDA approval for acute mania and for maintenance treatment. Olanzapine, in combination with fluoxetine, has recently received FDA approval for treatment of acute bipolar depression (see below).

There are concerns over sustained use of olanzapine due to safety and tolerability issues, particularly related to weight gain and increase in total cholesterol.[98] These issues can be addressed through careful management such as monitoring blood levels and side effects.

Risperidone — Having recently received FDA approval for treatment of acute mania, this is the only atypical antipsychotic with an injectable, slow-absorbing intramuscular form currently available.[99-103]

Quetiapine — An atypical antipsychotic with FDA approval for use in acute mania, quetiapine has been found effective for euphoric hypomanic or manic symptoms.[104, 105] Recent studies also suggest antidepressant efficacy for acutely depressed patients with bipolar disorder (see page 41).

Ziprasidone — Two recent double-blind, placebo-controlled trials in acute mania support efficacy for this medication in bipolar disorder and led to recent FDA approval for treatment of acute mania.[106, 107]

Special Considerations for Using Atypical Antipsychotics (AAPs)

Increased risk for obesity and type 2 diabetes, which can be exacerbated by weight gain side effects of AAPs, suggests that monitoring of body weight, calculation of body mass index (BMI), and education about sound diet, nutrition, and exercise are important treatment components.[108]

At the 2004 Consensus Development Conference on Antipsychotic Drugs and Obesity and Diabetes, experts from the American Diabetes Association, American Psychiatric Association, Association of Clinical Endocrinologists, and the North American Association for the Study of Obesity proposed a monitoring protocol for patients taking atypical antipsychotic medications. The table below illustrates the protocol:[109]

Monitoring Protocol for Patients Taking Atypical Antipsychotics*

Screening Measures	Baseline	4 Weeks	8 Weeks	12 Weeks	Quarterly	Annually	Every 5 Years
Personal/family history	X					X	
Weight (BMI)	X	X	X	X	X		
Waist circumference	X			X		X	
Blood pressure	X			X		X	
Fasting plasma glucose	X			X		X	
Fasting lipid profile	X			X			X

* More frequent assessments may be warranted based on clinical status.[109]

Research is underway to determine whether or not there is a direct effect of AAPs on metabolism separate from secondary effects due to weight gain.

Using Combination Medications

Combination therapy typically includes selections of medications from different drug classes, most notably lithium, anticonvulsants, and atypical antipsychotic medications.

Typically, published algorithms for treatment of bipolar disorder have recommended trying a single medication first, and then, if needed, combining medications.[74, 110–112] Newer guidelines recommend starting with combination medications for those whose symptoms are more severe.[73, 76] The majority of patients with bipolar disorder will need more than one medication to achieve mood stability. Recent studies support that the use of two medications to treat acute mania may increase the degree of response for many patients in the first three weeks of treatment.

What Medications are used to Treat Depression in Patients with Bipolar Disorder?

Medications used to treat depression in patients with bipolar disorder typically include lithium and the anticonvulsant lamotrigine as well as antidepressants [e.g., selective seratonin reuptake inhibitors (SSRIs), monoamine oxidase inhibitors (MAOIs), and others as listed in figure 3.5 on page 40]. Recently, a new combination preparation became the first medication to be FDA indicated for bipolar depression. An atypical antipsychotic has shown efficacy as well, with new research on this class likely to define a future role for these medications in bipolar depression treatment.

Although lithium monotherapy has some efficacy for treating depressive symptoms in patients with bipolar disorder, it is not as commonly used as other agents. Lithium may have notable protective effects in that it may minimize likelihood of self-harm.[120] To what degree this is a special property of lithium or due to more effective mood stabilization is unknown.

Prescribing an antidepressant to add to the patient's bipolar disorder medication regimen involves some risk of inducing a "switch" into mania.[121-125] However, this risk is fairly low with typically prescribed antidepressants (about 5–12 percent) compared to placebo when used as *add-on treatment.*[126, 127.]

Importantly, patients need to be aware that virtually all medications used to treat depression will require two to three weeks to see an improvement of symptoms. Often those around the individual experiencing depression will see improvement before the patient does.

Antidepressants are generally started following remission of manic symptoms if depression develops or if a patient was euthymic (not manic or depressed) and develops new depressive symptoms. If a person is experiencing mood instability or rapid cycling, use of antidepressants may actually worsen or prolong the period of instability. Balancing mood stabilizers must be done on a case-by-case basis, weighing the relative risks and benefits for the individual patient.

Optimal medication treatment for depressive symptoms is usually accomplished through the combination of:[128, 129]

▶ Lithium,

▶ Anticonvulsant medications (especially lamotrigine), which is taken once daily and generally well tolerated. It has little impact on sexual functioning or *body habitus,*

▶ Antidepressant medications.

A number of studies conclude that lithium may be effective for treatment of depression in persons with bipolar disorder.[113–117] *However, standard of care is usually to use lithium in combination with another agent. In a recent 18-month, double-blind maintenance trial, lithium was found to be more effective at preventing new manic than depressed episodes.*[118, 119]

add-on treatment — the addition of a new medication to already ongoing treatment

Figure 3.5 on the following page summarizes medications used to treat acute bipolar depression, including recommended dosages and side effects.

Antidepressant discontinuation should be done gradually unless there is a medical need to abruptly stop, such as intolerable side effects.

habitus — body build, can refer to weight impact of medications

Figure 3.5　Medication Dosages and Common Side Effects for Treating Acute Phase Depression in Patients with Bipolar Disorder

Type/Class: Medication*	Usual Target Dose**	Usual Maximum Recommended Dose (level)	Recommended Administration Schedule	Common Side Effects
Lithium (also available in a slow-absorption formula)	0.6–1.0 mEq/L	1.2 mEq/L	2 times daily or at bedtime	Tremor, drowsiness, nausea/vomiting, increased urine output, muscle weakness, thirst, dry mouth, cognitive impairment
Anticonvulsant: Lamotrigine**	200	600 mg/day	once daily	Headache, nausea, rash, dizziness, ataxia, somnolence, rhinitus
SSRIs:				Dizziness, dry mouth, insomnia, agitation, nausea, sexual dysfunction, headache
Citalopram	20–40	60 mg/day	once daily	
Escitalopram	10–20	20 mg/day	once daily	
Fluoxetine	20	80 mg/day	once daily	
Fluvoxamine	150–250	250 mg/day	once daily	
Paroxetine	20–50	60 mg/day	once daily	
Sertraline	100	200 mg/day	once daily	
Other Antidepressants:				
Bupropion	300	450 mg/day	2–3 times daily	Headache, agitation, weight loss, insomnia, nausea
Trazodone	300–600	600 mg/day	2–3 times daily	Dizziness, somnolence, insomnia, decreased appetite, anxiety, headache, nausea, sexual dysfunction, potential elevation in blood pressure at higher doses
Venlafaxine	150	375 mg/day	once daily	
Atypical Antipsychotics: Olanzapine and Fluoxetine	6–25	12–50 mg/day	at bedtime	See SSRIs (above) and olanzapine, quetiapine (figure 3.3 on page 33)
Quetiapine	300–600	800 mg/day	at bedtime	
MAOIs: Phenelzine	15	15–60 mg/day	1–2 times daily	Restlessness, dizziness, blurred vision, diarrhea, insomnia, weakness, irregular heart beat, headache, sexual dysfunction, weight loss/gain
Tranylcypromine	30	30–60 mg/day	once daily	Necessary to follow a diet eliminating tyramine, including cheese and red wine to avoid a hypertensive crisis; consult comprehensive list prior to initiation
Isocarboxazid	20	20–60 mg/day	once daily	

*This review focuses on commonly used medications and upcoming changes, but is neither comprehensive nor intended to provide prescription information. A physician or appropriate individual should be consulted prior to changing medications. Side effects may be less with slow-absorption forms of medications. Maximum daily doses often lower for slow-absorption forms relative to short-acting ones. For full information about medications, physicians should carefully review package inserts for individual medications or access the *Physicians Desk Reference*.

**It is important to follow initial dosing and rate of titration instructions listed on manufacturer package inserts.

Lamotrigine

Lamotrigine, an anticonvulsant has FDA approval for maintenance treatment to decrease the likelihood of new manic or depressed episodes in recently stabilized patients with bipolar I disorder. It is particularly effective in decreasing the likelihood of new depressive episodes. The drug has a rare, potential side effect of medically serious rashes (Stevens Johnson Syndrome or toxic epidermal necrolysis). This risk is strongly associated with *absolute starting dose* and/or *rate of initial titration*. Thus, following the recommended medication-dosing schedule is critical.

Antidepressant Medications

Antidepressant medications should not be added until the patient's primary medication dosing has decreased or eliminated symptoms of mania or hypomania. If used, there is little data to distinguish the effectiveness of using one type of antidepressant over another, so virtually all antidepressants listed below are used in bipolar disorder treatment. Antidepressants typically used for treating patients with bipolar disorder include:

► **SSRI medications**, which enhance serotonergic transmission, are in wide-spread clinical use and are administered as a single, daily dose, which potentially enhances compliance.

► **Bupropion** has little side-effect impact on sexual functioning, relatively few drug interactions, and has reasonable tolerability.

► **Trazodone**, not used as commonly for depression, is used in low dose to help problems with sleep.

► **Venlafaxine** is an antidepressant that enhances both noradrenergic and serotonergic neurotransmitters, usually used twice daily.

Atypical Antipsychotics

The FDA-approved combination of olanzapine-fluoxetine HCL for treatment of bipolar depression provides three dose formulations. Because olanzapine is a recognized antimanic agent, using this combination requires no additional antimanic medication unless a particular patient needs this to maintain mood stability.

Based on a recent, large-scale study, quetiapine appears to be significantly more effective than placebo for treating bipolar depression.[132] Further studies are underway to confirm these results.

absolute starting dose — amount of medication given when the patient first takes it

rate of initial titration — the rate by which a medication is increased to what is believed to be a minimum effective dose

Continuing controversy exists as to the long-term use of antidepressants with mood stabilizers in those with bipolar I disorder.[130] Research is underway to study the relative risks and benefits of this approach.[131]

Side-effect profile and clinical response varies among antidepressants; multiple trials may be necessary to find the best medication for a given individual.

Refer to the information on page 38 regarding special considerations for atypical antipsychotics.

Monoamine Oxidase Inhibitors (MAOIs)

MAOIs require all foods with tyramine be eliminated from the diet, including cheeses, fermented meats, red wine, and others. A comprehensive list should be consulted when using these medications. Diet restriction guidelines should be provided to all patients receiving MAOI medications.

These antidepressant drugs inhibit the monoamine oxidase enzyme in the central nervous system, intestinal tract, and platelets. This enzyme is linked to norepinephrine, a neurotransmitter implicated in the development of depression. However, because of potential health risks due to the risk of a hypertensive crisis (very high abrupt change in blood pressure) if the wrong foods are eaten and the special resulting dietary/medication restrictions, MAOIs are typically used only:

▶ After other treatments have failed

▶ When safety risks have been thoroughly evaluated

Tricyclic Antidepressants

These medications can also be effective for treating bipolar depression; however, they have more side effects and can be lethal in overdose. Tricyclics are considered an acceptable treatment strategy for patients with a prior history of good response and no ill effects to these medications.

Using a Treatment Algorithm for Depression in Bipolar Patients

For more information about the specific medications recommended in the TIMA 2005 treatment algorithms, refer to TIMA: Update to the Algorithms for Treatment of Bipolar I Disorder.[73]

Published treatment guidelines rank evidence-based options for treatment of bipolar depression. The recently revised TIMA guideline, shown in figure 3.6 on the next page, provides one such example.[73]

This algorithm clearly delineates between treatment approaches for patients who do and do not have a history of severe mania. This is especially important because lamotrigine, which has efficacy for treating bipolar depression, has limited antimanic efficacy and, in combination with an antidepressant, may require the addition of an antimanic agent to prevent mood switch.[133]

Recent studies with atypical antipsychotic agents support a role for their use in treatment of bipolar depression. Further studies are also underway to confirm these findings. Studies are also underway to assess the antidepressant potential of other atypical agents. Earlier safety considerations on the use of atypical antipsychotics apply here.

Figure 3.6 TIMA Algorithm for Treating Bipolar I Disorder, Currently Depressed (2005)

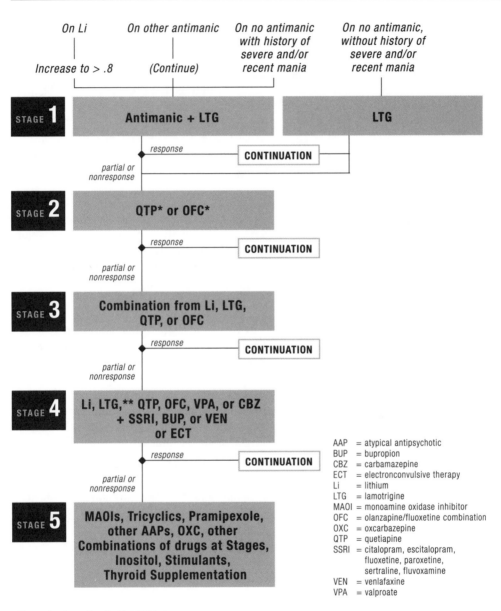

On Li

Increase to > .8

On other antimanic

(Continue)

On no antimanic with history of severe and/or recent mania

On no antimanic, without history of severe and/or recent mania

STAGE 1 — Antimanic + LTG | LTG

response → CONTINUATION

partial or nonresponse

STAGE 2 — QTP* or OFC*

response → CONTINUATION

partial or nonresponse

STAGE 3 — Combination from Li, LTG, QTP, or OFC

response → CONTINUATION

partial or nonresponse

STAGE 4 — Li, LTG,** QTP, OFC, VPA, or CBZ + SSRI, BUP, or VEN or ECT

response → CONTINUATION

partial or nonresponse

STAGE 5 — MAOIs, Tricyclics, Pramipexole, other AAPs, OXC, other Combinations of drugs at Stages, Inositol, Stimulants, Thyroid Supplementation

AAP = atypical antipsychotic
BUP = bupropion
CBZ = carbamazepine
ECT = electronconvulsive therapy
Li = lithium
LTG = lamotrigine
MAOI = monoamine oxidase inhibitor
OFC = olanzapine/fluoxetine combination
OXC = oxcarbazepine
QTP = quetiapine
SSRI = citalopram, escitalopram, fluoxetine, paroxetine, sertraline, fluvoxamine
VEN = venlafaxine
VPA = valproate

*Note safety issue described in TIMA text.

**LTG has limited antimanic efficacy and, in combination with an antidepressant, may require the addition of an antimanic.

Effectiveness of Medications for Treating Depression in Bipolar Disorder

A number of studies conclude that lithium may be effective for treatment of depression in persons with bipolar disorder.[113-117] However, standard of care is usually to use lithium in combination with another agent. In a recent 18-month, double-blind maintenance trial, lithium was found to be more effective at preventing new manic than depressed episodes.[118, 119]

There is remarkably little data on treatment of depression in bipolar disorder, and most treatment recommendations are based on expert consensus and common clinical practice rather than scientifically rigorous studies. Research has been done on lithium, lamotrigine, SSRIs, and other antidepressants for treating bipolar depression. A recent study led to FDA approval of an olanzapine-fluoxetine combination. Another study has been completed supporting the use of quetiapine as well. However, as with all medication choices, a balance of efficacy and tolerability must be considered. There are tremendous individual differences in response and sensitivity to side effects in all medications discussed.

Lamotrigine

Two blinded studies support lamotrigine's efficacy for treatment of bipolar depression.[133, 134] This was the first medication since lithium in the 1970s to receive FDA approval for maintenance treatment to decrease the likelihood of new manic or depressed episodes in recently stabilized patients with bipolar I disorder.[118, 119]

SSRIs

Because medication responsiveness and side effects differ from one individual to another, and because treatments developed and proven safe for other disorders may offer some benefits, it is important to work closely with each patient to optimize their medications.

Limited controlled evidence exists for using SSRIs to treat bipolar depression.[135-138] It is important to use these medications in combination with an antimanic agent to prevent bipolar "switch."

Atypical Antipsychotics

Further study is needed to determine to what extent atypical antipsychotics have specific antidepressant efficacy in addition to their demonstrated antimanic efficacy.

Olanzapine-Fluoxetine Combination — A recent placebo-controlled study in patients with bipolar I disorder currently depressed found significant efficacy for the combination of olanzapine (an atypical antipsychotic) and fluoxetine (an SSRI) without on increased risk for development of mania.[139] In this study, the use of olanzapine alone was also significant relative to placebo, although the results were not as striking nor of the same effect size as the combination.

For more information on special considerations for using atypical antipsychotics, see page 38.

Quetiapine — A recent, large study of people suffering from acute bipolar depression found that quetiapine was significantly more effective than placebo. However, 26 percent of those receiving 600 mg/day of the drug dropped out of the study due to side effects. Similarly, 16 percent of those receiving 300 mg/day dropped out prematurely.[132]

MAOIs (tranylcypromine) — Studies on the use of MAOIs support their effectiveness for treatment of major depressive episodes in bipolar disorder.[140-142]

Tricyclic Antidepressants — Despite numerous disadvantages, tricyclic antidepressant medications can also be effective for treating bipolar depression.[124, 142-144]

What Strategies are Recommended for Maintenance Treatment?

There are relatively few scientific studies on the long-term management of patients with bipolar disorder. In practice, virtually all patients will need ongoing anti-manic medication to prevent symptom relapse. For those taking a combination of mood stabilizers and making medication changes, the clinician should taper one medication either associated with side effects or limited partial response, while continuing other medications. Current general practice guidelines indicate the use of lifetime treatment following two manic episodes, or one episode if severe and/or a significant family history of bipolar or major depressive disorder exists.

Maintenance should involve the lowest possible dose that will achieve ongoing mood stabilization.

Clinicians and patients need to carefully collaborate on the initiation and duration of maintenance pharmacological management of those with bipolar disorder. Key issues to resolve are:

- ▶ Patient personal preference and response
- ▶ Risk factors for recurrence
- ▶ Side-effect profile
- ▶ Patient ability to tolerate the prescribed medication (critical to compliance)

Current recommendations are to gradually taper antidepressant treatment following symptom remission and after a period of stability lasting two to four months. However, some patients with bipolar disorder may need ongoing antidepressant treatment along with antimanic agents.[131] As early as the 1970s, researchers noticed that sometimes medications necessary for minimizing manic symptoms pushed the brain below a euthymic level, thus necessitating use of antidepressants to balance the brain chemistry.

Effectiveness of Maintenance Treatment for Bipolar Patients

New research addresses using lithium, lamotrigine, aripiprazole, and olanzapine for maintenance treatment. As of 2004, these medications are FDA approved for maintenance treatment. All of the studies leading to FDA approval were completed with patients with bipolar I disorder. As discussed elsewhere in this book, the data to guide treatment decisions for patients with bipolar II disorder are very limited. Because of this, treatment algorithms that are evidence-based, such as presented here, are specific for patients with bipolar I disorder. The degree to which these treatments and combinations will apply for BD-II is a critically needed area of research.

Lithium — Many years ago, the FDA approved the use of lithium to prevent new episodes. Lithium has some efficacy to decrease depressive symptoms, but is not used as commonly for this as other agents. Recent research indicates that lithium may minimize the likelihood of self-harm; however, it is unknown whether this is a special property of the drug or due to effective mood stabilization.[120]

Lamotrigine — In June 2003, lamotrigine received FDA approval for prevention of mood episodes of all types in bipolar disorder, making it the first anticonvulsant to receive this approval.[118, 119]

Carbamazepine — A recent, open-label study found that an extended-release formulation of carbamazepine was effective for maintenance treatment for those experiencing recently manic/mixed symptoms.[145]

Atypical Antipsychotics — Based on a recent set of studies, an atypical antipsychotic, olanzapine, has received FDA approval for maintenance treatment. Physicians and patients should discuss the relative risks and benefits of long-term use of olanzapine, given the safety concerns. Olanzapine has shown efficacy in preventing new manic symptoms.[98, 146, 147]

Aripiprazole was found superior to placebo in a six-month trial following stabilization.[148] This medication plus quetiapine, risperidone, and ziprasidone are all recommended for maintenance treatment of bipolar disorder; however, much research on maintenance use of these drugs to date comes from open, uncontrolled studies of these in combination with other established medications. More research is also needed to determine safety.

Clozapine has proven some effectiveness for maintenance treatment in recent studies, and is recommended for treatment-resistant patients but requires ongoing monitoring for adverse events.[91, 109, 145]

Antidepressants — For antidepressants, no definitive research exists to resolve maintenance issues. On one hand, recent major guidelines recommend stopping antidepressants within a few weeks or months after resolution of depressive symptoms.[110, 111, 149] However, a recent retrospective study suggests that those patients who continue to take an antidepressant for one year (in combination with an anti-manic medication) following a depressive episode have fewer clinical symptoms, function better, and are not at a higher risk for manic switch.[131] This important, new data needs to be addressed in randomized prospective study to clarify the long-term management for patients recently depressed.

Figure 3.7 TIMA Recommendations for Bipolar Disorder Maintenance Treatment, Most Recent Episode Manic, Mixed, Hypomanic (2005)

It is an option to remain on well-tolerated, effective, acute phase treatments. Available evidence supports the following options for prevention of new episodes or maintenance treatment.

Level **I**

For those with a history of frequent, recent, or severe mania, Lithium or Valproate is recommended. For those without frequent, recent, or severe mania, Lithium, Valproate, or Lamotrigine are acceptable choices. An alternative is Olanzapine.[a]

Level **II**

Aripiprazole[b]

Level **III**

Carbamazepine or Clozapine[a]

Level **IV**

Quetiapine,[b] Risperidone,[b] or Ziprasidone[b]

Level **V**

Typical antipsychotics,[a] Oxcarbazepine,[b] ECT

[a]Safety issues warrant careful consideration of this option for long-term use.

[b]Relatively limited information is currently available on these agents in long-term use.

Figure 3.8   TIMA Recommendations for Bipolar Disorder Maintenance Treatment, Most Recent Episode Depressed (2005)

It is an option to remain on well-tolerated, effective, acute phase treatments. Available evidence supports the following options for maintenance treatment.

Level I

Lamotrigine is recommended in combination with an antimanic agent for those with recent and/or severe history of mania. For all others, Lamotrigine monotherapy is a reasonable maintenance treatment.

Level II

Lithium

Level III

Combination of an antimanic and antidepressant that has been effective in the past, including Olanzapine-Fluoxetine Combination.[a]

Level IV

Valproate, Carbamazepine, Aripiprazole,[b] Clozapine,[a] Olanzapine,[a] Quetiapine,[b] Risperidone,[b] Ziprasidone[b]

Level V

Typical antipsychotics, Oxcarbazepine, ECT

[a]Safety issues warrant careful consideration of this option for potential long-term use.

[b]Relatively limited information is currently available on these agents in long-term use.

How Can Medication Treatment of Side Effects be Managed?

Key side effects that patients with bipolar disorder may experience with medication therapy include gastrointestinal upset, tremor, sedation, extrapyramidal symptoms (Parkinson-like side effects, such as flat facial expression, stiff muscles, and slowed movements), tardive dyskinesia (development of involuntary motor movements, which may persist beyond use of the medication — usually associated with older antipsychotics), insomnia, and sexual dysfunction.

A key clinical treatment issue in managing patients' medications is **how** changes are made. Always overlap a new medication with ongoing medications, and gradually taper any medication being discontinued unless there is a medical necessity to rapidly stop (e.g., allergic reaction or severe side effects). Figure 3.9 on the next page provides an at-a-glance view of medication trade names. For full information about medications, physicians should carefully review package inserts for individual medications or access the *Physicians Desk Reference*.

Another critical aspect of managing side effects is monitoring for potential drug interactions. Drugs taken for heart, renal, endocrinologic, or hepatic disease may interact with a mood stabilizer like lithium or other antimanic/antidepressive medications. Patients should be questioned about over-the-counter medication use as well.

*Figure 3.10, on the page 51 presents a summary of recommendations compiled from the **Physicians Desk Reference** and the TMAP Handbook for these side effects. This list is neither comprehensive nor intended to replace medical evaluation of side effects, but provides a general example of some of the more usual approaches to side effects in this population.*

Clinicians need to carefully discuss both response and side effects with patients, emphasizing that, for the vast majority of patients, bipolar disorder requires lifelong treatment.

How are Electroconvulsive Therapy (ECT) and Alternative Medicine Used to Treat Patients with Bipolar Disorder?

ECT is an accepted, effective treatment for acute mania as well as for depression, whether in patients with bipolar or unipolar disorder.[150, 151] However, safety, tolerability, and patient acceptance issues typically rank ECT behind pharmacological approaches. Due to the range of medications now available, ECT is reserved for patients unresponsive to or unable to take current medications, women who are pregnant, and patients in acute danger of committing suicide or who suffer dangerous lack of food and fluid intake due to severe depressive symptoms. The response to this treatment is quite rapid, with striking improvements seen often within one to two weeks.

In addition to ECT, less-invasive techniques, such as magnetic stimulation of an *epileptic seizure* and *vagal nerve stimulation* are now being explored. In epileptic seizures, impacts range from a

epileptic seizure — an uncontrolled discharge of brain cells

vagal nerve stimulation — an FDA-approved treatment for refractory epilepsy and depression now being explored for bipolar disorder

full, grand mal seizure associated with brief loss of consciousness and bladder control to a partial seizure where aberrant, excitable neural activity stays localized. Manifestations of partial seizures are extensive and can range from isolated limb movements to temporary blindness. In vagal nerve stimulation, a pacemaker is inserted and a wire wrapped around the vagus nerve in the neck, which is then stimulated by a small electrical current every few minutes. The mechanism of efficacy is unknown.

Other alternative therapies are currently being studied, including adjunctive treatments using fish oils (Omega 3), acupuncture, and mineral supplements. Although researchers anticipate new developments from these studies, caution should be exercised before embracing alternative or complementary approaches. For example, Kava Kava (an herb sometimes used to combat anxiety) has recently been associated with cases of liver failure.[152]

Figure 3.9   Trade Names for Common Bipolar Medications

Medication	Trade Name (s)	Medication	
Lithium	Eskalith,® Lithobid®		

Anticonvulsants

Medication	Trade Name (s)	Medication	
Carbamazepine	Equetro,™ Tegretol,® Carbatrol®	Topiramate	Topamax®
Gabapentin	Neurontin®	Valproate	Depakote,® Depakene®
Lamotrigine	Lamictal®		

Antidepressants

Medication	Trade Name (s)	Medication	
Amitriptyline	Elavil,® Endep®	Maprotiline	Ludiomil®
Amoxapine	Ascendin®	Mirtazapine	Remeron®
Bupropion	Wellbutrin®	Nortriptyline	Aventyl,® Pamelor®
Citalopram	Celexa®	Paroxetine	Paxil®
Clomipramine	Anafranil®	Protriptyline	Vivactil®
Desipramine	Norpramin®	Sertraline	Zoloft®
Doxepin	Adapin,® Sinequan®	Trazodone	Desyrel®
Fluoxetine	Prozac®	Trimipramine	Surmontil®
Fluvoxamine	Luvox®	Venlafaxine	Effexor®
Imipramine	Tofranil®		

Atypical Antipsychotics

Medication	Trade Name (s)	Medication	
Aripiprazole	Abilify®	Quetiapine	Seroquel®
Clozapine	Clozaril®	Risperidone	Risperdal®
Olanzapine	Zyprexa®	Ziprasidone	Geodon®

MAOIs

Medication	Trade Name (s)	Medication	
Isocarboxazid	Marplan®	Selegiline	Eldepryl®
Phenelzine	Nardil®	Tranylcypromine	Parnate®

Figure 3.10   Treating Bipolar Disorder Medication Side Effects

Side Effects	Recommendations
GI Upset	• Administer medication with food and large quantities of liquid. • Consider lowering dose, if possible. • Use sustained-release preparations of medications when available. • Some data suggest that this side effect can be successfully treated with H2 blockers (e.g., cimetidine, ranitidine).
Tremor	**Enhanced physiologic tremor — A fine tremor of approximately 8–10 Hz.; made worse when hands are outstretched** • Check blood levels of medication. • Decrease dose, divide dose, or change to slow-absorption preparation of the medication. • Propranolol can be given at 20–30 mg, 3 times daily, or 80 mg long-acting, daily. **Parkinsonian tremor — Coarse tremor at rest of approximately 4–6 Hz.** • Decrease dose, divide dose, use bedtime dosing, or switch to alternate medication. • Pharmacological treatments include benztropine 1–2 mg twice daily, amantadine 100 mg, 2 or 3 times daily, and diphenhydramine 25–50 mg, 2 or 3 times daily.
Sedation	• Change to bedtime dosing. • Substitute a less-sedating, alternative medication.
Extra-pyramidal Symptoms (EPS)	• This is usually seen with older antipsychotics. • Treat tremor as suggested above. • Reduce dose of antipsychotic medication. • Akathisia may respond to propranolol 20–30 mg, 3 times a day (or 80 mg slow-absorbing form, daily), benztropine, amantadine, or diphenhydramine. If ineffective, alternatives include clonidine (0.1 mg, 3 times a day) and lorazepam (1–2 mg, 2–3 times daily). • Dystonic reactions can often be prevented by benztropine 1 mg 2 or 3 times daily for the first few days of antipsychotic therapy. Acute dystonic reactions are generally managed with benztropine 1–2 mg or lorazepam 1 mg intramuscular.
Tardive Dyskinesia (TD)	• Prescribe antipsychotics in the lowest dose necessary for the shortest time possible. • Consider alternatives for mood stabilization and control of agitation. • Use atypical antipsychotic medications, which appear to have a lower incidence of TD. • Some evidence that vitamin E given in high doses (>1,000 units per day) may decrease some symptoms of TD for some patients.
Insomnia	• Use morning dosing, or spread total daily dose as early in the day as possible. • Use QHS dosing for any potentially sedating medications. • Use zolpidem (5–10 mg) at bedtime, zaleplon (5–20 mg; 10 mg recommended dose) at bedtime, or benzodiazepine, such as temazepam (15–30 mg) at night. Antipsychotics should always be considered second- or third-line agents for insomnia due to their risk of extrapyramidal symptoms and tardive dyskinesia. Avoid use of higher doses of trazodone for sleep as it is an antidepressant and thus has the potential for destabilizing and increasing symptoms of mania in patients with bipolar disorder. Benzodiazepines are best avoided in patients with prior history of substance abuse/dependence or who are at risk for substance abuse. Nonaddicting agents are preferred.
Sexual Dysfunction	• Add yohimbine at 4–7.5 mg, 3 times a day, cyproheptadine at 4–8 mg given shortly before sexual intercourse, or the antidepressant bupropion given at dosages of 75–300 mg per day. Bupropion has the advantage of potentially also augmenting the antidepressant efficacy of the SSRI.

How Does Comorbidity Impact Medication Treatment for Bipolar Disorder?

Bipolar disorder is the psychiatric illness most associated with or most likely to have comorbid diagnoses, which include:[15]

- ▶ Alcohol and/or substance abuse or dependence (lifetime prevalence) — over 50 percent of those with bipolar disorder
- ▶ Anxiety disorders (e.g., panic, general anxiety, obsessive-compulsive, and post-traumatic stress disorders) — 20 to 40 percent of those with bipolar disorder
- ▶ Eating disorders
- ▶ Impulse dyscontrol disorders

Key Concepts for Chapter Three:

1. Bipolar disorder is a medical-biological illness, related to changes in brain activity, with a genetic component.

2. Treatment for bipolar disorder must include mood stabilizing medications.

3. For hypomania/mania, classes of medications used include lithium, anticonvulsants, and atypical antipsychotics; a balanced treatment approach must consider efficacy, tolerability, and safety data.

4. Combination treatment is recommended at the outset for treating more severe symptoms, regardless of the phase of the illness.

5. Maintenance treatment is recommended for all patients diagnosed with bipolar I disorder.

6. It is important to treat the depressive phase of the illness because of the potential for suicide; however, never use an antidepressant alone without a mood stabilizing agent.

7. Medications used to treat bipolar disorder often cause side effects, which must be minimized to maintain adherence to treatment.

8. Medication changes should be done using an overlap-and-taper strategy unless medical necessity requires abrupt discontinuation.

Chapter 4:
Psychosocial Treatments for Bipolar Disorder

This chapter answers the following:

▶ **Why Add Psychosocial Interventions to Pharmacotherapy?** — This section discusses psychosocial therapy's adjunctive treatment role for improving medication adherence, coping with stress, preventing relapse, and improving functioning and quality of life.

▶ **What Psychosocial Interventions are most Successful for Treating Bipolar Disorder?** — This section presents an overview of the types of successful interventions used as adjunct therapy to medication.

▶ **What is the Psychoeducational Approach to Bipolar Disorder Treatment?** — This section covers key psychoeducational treatment strategies, the TMAP package, and psychoeducation effectiveness.

▶ **What is Family-Focused Treatment (FFT) for Bipolar Disorder?** — This section covers FFT (psychoeducation, communication awareness, and problem-solving skills) as well as results of recent efficacy studies.

▶ **What Individual Psychosocial Approaches are used to Treat Bipolar Disorder?** — This section reviews cognitive-behavioral therapy (CBT) and interpersonal social rhythm therapy (IPSRT). Results of efficacy studies follow each treatment discussion.

P SYCHOLOGICAL treatments for bipolar disorder have evolved over the years. Initially, psychosocial therapy was the only clinical option for treatment of bipolar disorder. As effective medication treatments became available, interest in developing psychosocial treatments and research into the efficacy of these interventions waned. While there is increased recognition that bipolar disorder is a "brain disease" requiring pharmacological treatment, psychological therapies are potentially important and useful adjuncts to that primary treatment. Today, psychosocial interventions, including psychoeducation and more traditional therapies, once again play an important role in treating bipolar disorder.

Efficacy research for psychosocial treatments is limited; many studies that currently exist are not well controlled, are not large enough, or do not address long-term outcomes.

Why Add Psychosocial Interventions to Pharmacotherapy?

Both psychosocial therapy outcome studies and published treatment guidelines support the use of psychosocial treatment approaches as a possible adjunct to pharmacological therapy.

According to recent reviews of psychosocial therapy outcome studies in bipolar disorder, psychoeducational and cognitive-behavioral strategies (included as adjunct to traditional pharmacological treatments) result in a decreased rate of hospitalization and incidence of relapse as well as improved medication adherence and overall clinical symptoms.[153–155]

Longitudinal data collected in the 1990s suggest that those with bipolar disorder suffer relapse at rates as high as 40 percent (year one), 60 percent (year two), and 73 percent (years 5+).[153]

53

Published guidelines for treating bipolar disorder also support the use of psychosocial interventions. For example, the "Expert Consensus Guideline" for bipolar disorder endorses mood-stabilizing medication as the first line of treatment for depression in bipolar disorder, but includes alternative options of either treatment with an antidepressant medication or addition of psychosocial therapy to existing medication.[110]

A variety of research studies have looked at the link between psychosocial variables (e.g., *expressed emotion* in families, negative life events, and dysfunctional attitudes and *attributional styles*) and course of a person's bipolar illness. These studies found **increased**:

expressed emotion — critical, hostile, and overemotional communication patterns

attributional styles — one's tendencies in making causal explanations about a variety of intra- and interpersonal events in their lives

- ▶ Relapse rates in families with high expressed emotion
- ▶ Recovery time for those experiencing negative life events
- ▶ Likelihood for a person to develop affective symptoms among those with maladaptive ways of thinking about themselves and others and those suffering environmental stress
- ▶ New episodes among those suffering disrupted sleep-wake schedules, often triggered by negative life events and the person's difficulty coping effectively with those events

Evidence suggests that psychosocial therapy may be helpful for individuals with bipolar disorder by improving adherence to treatment, helping develop better coping mechanisms to deal with stressful life events, preventing relapse, and generally improving functioning and quality of life.

Psychosocial treatments for bipolar disorder tend to focus on the management of life circumstances that impact how one expresses and deals with the disorder.[156, 157]

Improving Adherence to Medication Treatment

Despite advances in effective medication treatments for bipolar disorder, some people's symptoms do not completely remit or disappear. Only about 50–60 percent of acutely ill patients respond to lithium or anticonvulsants alone, and many require combinations of drugs, as described in chapter three. As medication combinations become more complex, the likelihood of side effects (e.g., weight gain, nausea, cognitive "dullness") increases and patients' willingness to comply with prescribed regimens decreases. Key reasons for patients to lapse or totally stop taking their medications include:

Although hypomanic symptoms may be appealing, adhering to a prescribed medication treatment plan is critical. Untreated hypomania may lead to mania in those with bipolar I disorder, and often to poor decision making that damages relationships, financial stability, physical health, or employment security.

- ▶ Not wanting to lose what many patients perceive as the more satisfying and productive symptom spectrum, which makes side effects even more intolerable
- ▶ Finding the negative side effects of some medications intolerable

▶ Mistakenly thinking that, by not experiencing an episode in some time, they have been "cured" and no longer require treatment

Research indicates that, in the first year of treatment, one-half to two-thirds of patients fail to comply with medication treatment. Some data suggests that most patients only remain fully compliant with mood stabilizing medication for two months.[158-161]

Optimum treatment of bipolar disorder occurs when psychosocial interventions augment pharmacological treatments. Several studies suggest that psychoeducation and interventions that address medication compliance substantially improve adherence to treatment and clinical and functional outcomes.

Because of these issues, psychosocial interventions for bipolar disorder emphasize education on the recurrent and life-long nature of this illness and the importance of medication compliance.

> *Discontinuing medications, particularly without physician supervision, carries the risk of relapse, diminished response to future treatments, and a more severe course of illness.*
>
> *Clinicians and patients should work together to find a treatment plan that is acceptable, and not "settle" for something with undesired side effects that may eventually justify noncompliance.*

Coping with Stress

Psychosocial therapy can help patients deal with both the environmental and psychological factors that contribute to episode frequency and the rate of recovery from mood episodes. Evidence suggests that new episodes can be prompted by:[162-164]

▶ Stressful life events

▶ Activities that disrupt the sleep/wake rhythms (working swing shifts or jet lag), which can prompt a manic episode

▶ Psychological factors, such as how one's attributional style and attitudes may interact with life events to predict increased symptoms

An example of an attributional style might be attributing negative life events (e.g., being laid off from a seasonal job) in terms of dispositional characteristics (e.g., "I was terrible on the cash register and made too many mistakes."). The person may experience more depressive symptoms than those who attribute the same event to external causes (e.g., "They don't need me anymore because the holiday rush is over.").

People with chronic bipolar disorder may have limited social support, which can negatively impact their response to treatment. Absence of social support (e.g., having few friends) predicts a longer time to recovery after a manic, depressed, or mixed episode as well as higher levels of depression over six months.[165]

Because of the connections between physical and environmental factors and course of illness, psychosocial interventions for patients with bipolar disorder might focus on:

▶ Increasing social support (e.g., working with the patient to improve existing relationships, or to establish and build new relationships)

▶ Teaching the importance of regulating sleep-wake cycles (e.g., working with the patient to establish a sleep "routine," such as going to bed by 11:00 p.m. each night and using an alarm clock to wake at a consistent hour), which may minimize the precipitation of mood shifts

▶ Teaching coping methods for stressful life events (e.g., assertive communication or relaxation techniques)

▶ Identifying and altering psychological mechanisms that exacerbate symptoms (e.g., a person's tendency to minimize symptoms and discontinue medications) and developing a strategy to correct that instinct

Preventing Relapse

Even during periods of adequate medication treatment and relatively stable moods, many individuals with bipolar disorder continue to experience significant functional impairment.[10, 12, 167]

Bipolar disorder is a lifetime condition characterized by repeated mood episodes. Despite previously adequate treatment, individuals can experience relapse, or the emergence of a new mood episode (depression, hypomania, mania, or mixed) after achieving remission. Psychosocial treatment may augment the effects of pharmacotherapy in preventing relapse by teaching patients and their loved ones to identify early warning signs that might signal an imminent episode. In general, as patients experience longer intervals of wellness, their risk of a new episode decreases.[166]

Along with recognition of the early warning signs, individuals should have a plan for dealing with them, including concrete actions one can quickly take to stabilize the situation, such as calling the clinician.

Individuals need to learn to recognize external events that may trigger an increase in symptoms (e.g., an upcoming family event that has been stressful in the past). Additionally, psychosocial treatment can help individuals learn to monitor themselves for unique behaviors that are reliable warning signs of an increase in symptoms or an emergent episode. These warning signs tend to be very unique for each individual, but can be identified, monitored, and acted upon as a helpful relapse prevention tool. For example, a patient might identify restless sleep, insomnia, increased irritability, or more frequent purchase of lottery tickets as key warning signs.

Finally, psychosocial treatment can help with relapse prevention by facilitating the development of a plan to promote wellness, such as regularly eating healthy meals, getting adequate sleep, limiting or avoiding alcohol, and exercising regularly.

Improving Functioning and Quality of Life

Even during periods of adequate medication treatment and relatively stable moods, many individuals with bipolar disorder continue to experience significant functional impairment.[10, 12, 167] At work, this ongoing occupational dysfunction is evident in the finding that six months after hospitalization, 30 percent of patients were unable to work at all, and only 21 percent worked at their expected level.[168] At home, bipolar disorder is associated with high rates of family or marital conflict, separation, and divorce.[12] Using psychosocial interventions to help develop coping skills for both manic and depressive symptoms may lessen the disorder's functional impact. Patients can learn to optimize their social and occupational functioning, while coping with the diagnosis and treatment of a chronic illness.

What Psychosocial Interventions are most Successful for Treating Bipolar Disorder?

In general, psychotherapeutic approaches that are seen as most beneficial for those with bipolar disorder are multifaceted, typically including psychoeducation, medication adherence, individual therapy, and marital and/or family involvement/therapy. Bauer and McBride (1996) describe key elements of psychosocial therapy of patients with bipolar disorder, summarized from descriptive reports of successful interventions.[169] The table on the next page (figure 4.1) presents a brief overview of these

From the Patient's Perspective

I'm really beginning to come to terms with what it means to have bipolar disorder. I don't think I really understood it in the beginning. It helps to have someone to talk with about having this illness, and to help me deal with some of the problems in my life. My husband is so angry with me for spending all the money, and I am trying to improve my communication skills so that he and I can get through this difficult time. I was also having such a hard time believing that this was something serious - I thought the doctor was just overreacting. But when I stopped my medication, I quickly figured out that these symptoms are serious, and they will come back if I don't take care of myself and follow my treatment plan.

Figure 4.1   Elements of Successful Psychological Interventions for Bipolar Disorder

Type of Intervention	Elements of Intervention	Examples of Strategies within Element
Psychoeducational Interventions	• Education regarding illness and treatment	Informational videos or written materials about bipolar disorder
	• Illness management skills	Teaching strategies to remind patients to take medications as prescribed, such as alarms, pillboxes, or charts; rehearsal of steps to take when symptoms increase; education regarding the importance of treatment adherence
Problem-Solving/Coping Interventions	• Work management	Interventions to assist patient in navigating work problems, such as negotiating for a leave of absence
	• Family management	Interventions to assist patient coping with family issues, such as a relative who insists their problems are "all in their head"
	• Life goals outside of illness	Interventions to help patient reach life goals, such as completing school applications or starting a new hobby
Psychodynamic/ Interpersonal Interventions	• Dealing with unstable interpersonal relationships	Interventions such as family or couple therapy to enhance relationship and communication with significant others
	• Coping with loss	Interventions that assist the patient to address and reduce feelings of grief and loss (may be loss due to death of a loved one, loss of plans and expectations set prior to illness, etc.)
	• Vulnerability	Interventions that assist the patient to develop resiliency and confidence
	• Self-concept	Interventions that assist the patient to develop a healthy and realistic sense of self

Adapted from Bauer M & McBride L, (1996).[169]

elements and offers some overall guidance on what psychosocial interventions may be included in a treatment "package" for a patient with bipolar disorder.

While research on psychosocial interventions for bipolar disorder is still limited, specific psychotherapies that have been shown to be effective for patients with bipolar disorder include:

▶ Psychoeducational Programs

▶ Family-Focused Treatment (FFT)

▶ Individual Treatments, such as Cognitive-Behavioral Therapy (CBT) and Interpersonal Social Rhythm Therapy (IPSRT)

What is the Psychoeducational Approach to Bipolar Disorder Treatment?

Psychoeducation involves teaching patients and their families, if possible, about bipolar disorder, treatment options, and how to recognize signs of relapse, so that they can get necessary treatment before their difficulty worsens or reoccurs. Additionally, those close to the patient may learn coping strategies and problem-solving skills to help them deal more effectively with their loved one with bipolar disorder. Current thinking regarding the role of psychosocial treatments for bipolar disorder emphasizes an integrative approach, where one might pick and choose a different focus of education depending on illness and patient characteristics. For example, if a patient demonstrates a persistent problem taking medications as directed, psychoeducation for that person may focus on developing tools to help them be more consistent (e.g., using a timer, pill box, or medication checklist posted in a prominent location in their home).

This section reviews the psychoeducational approach to treating bipolar disorder as well as treatment strategies and research on its efficacy when used as an adjunct to medication therapy.

Psychoeducational Treatment Strategies

Psychoeducational treatment strategies may focus on one or more of the following:

▶ **Taking prescribed medications as directed** — Helping the patient understand how medication compliance will improve symptoms and long-term course of illness, potentially prolonging periods of wellness between episodes, and reducing or minimizing mood symptoms when they do occur. Additionally, psychoeducation may include educating the patient about reasons people choose to discontinue medications and other treatments for bipolar disorder, and the possible consequences of that decision.

It is critical to educate patients and their families about adherence to medication treatment, including the benefits of taking medications and what side effects they may experience.

▶ **Understanding risk factors for relapse** — Patients will learn critical events or situations that make them more prone to relapse, for example, discontinuing medications, or experiencing particularly stressful life events, such as moving. With this knowledge and the awareness that these things may precipitate relapse, patients are more able to recognize and proactively respond if early symptoms emerge.

▶ **Recognizing warning signs of relapse** — Patients may learn to identify their own unique and individual warning signs that signal an emergent mood episode. For example, one individual may learn to recognize that sleeping greater than 10 hours per night usually occurs before the onset of a new depressive episode.

> ▶ **Managing stressful life events** — Helping the patient identify what life events can be particularly stressful and developing strategies (e.g., exercising, calling on supportive friends, or changing thought patterns) to better manage those events

> ▶ **Protective factors** — Patients may learn to identify protective factors in their lives that support their treatment and management of bipolar symptoms (e.g., having daily contact with a family member or participating in a support group of friends).

Psychoeducation can be simple and straightforward (a patient and nurse discussing a new medication) or more complex and multifaceted (structuring a psychoeducational "package" of written, visual, and interactive educational materials about the disorder and treatment). One such package was developed for use in the Texas Medication Algorithm Project (TMAP) and includes written materials, a video, pictures depicting important lessons, and instructions for an interactive, peer-led group experience.

The TMAP psychoeducational package is used in conjunction with medication guidelines for major depressive disorder, bipolar disorder, and schizophrenia.

The TMAP disease management approach includes:

> ▶ Evidence-based medication guidelines, such as the medication algorithms featured on pages 35 and 43 in chapter three

> ▶ Structured assessments (e.g., the IDS-SR, YMRS, and BPRS in chapter two and appendix B)

> ▶ Standardized clinical record keeping which includes routine clinical assessment instruments to enhance consistency and guide clinical decision making and treatment planning

In psychoeducational interventions, patients learn to recognize signs and symptoms of their illness and take steps to prevent onset of new episodes. One helpful tool may be the daily Life Chart, which can be used by the individual to monitor and track daily moods and gain insight into how these relate to critical life events. As a psychoeducational tool (rather than a diagnostic tool as noted in chapter two and appendix C), the Life Chart helps the patient learn to identify patterns in their moods and to track the relationship of life events to mood changes. For example, a patient may realize that they regularly experience increases in depressive symptoms at the time of their menses and can then strategize ways to anticipate and cope with these symptoms.

TMAP includes tools that provide patient and family education, address symptoms and treatment, and emphasize the development of a collaborative treatment relationship.[170] Access additional program information at: http://www.dshs.state.tx.us/mhprograms/TMAP.shtm.

Appendix C includes a sample of the Life Chart.

Effectiveness of Psychoeducation

Several published psychotherapeutic approaches, such as the Life Goals Program, include a psychoeducational component in the early phase of treatment and then introduce other, more sophisticated approaches as the patient's treatment progresses.[169]

A recent, blinded controlled study of a psychoeducational intervention included 120 patients with BD-I and BD-II.[171] Outpatients in remission continued to receive standard pharmacologic treatment, and in addition, completed either 21 sessions of group psychoeducation or non-structured group meetings. Psychoeducation was significantly better than the control condition in preventing recurrence of any mood episode (60 vs. 38 percent; $p<.05$ in the 20-week treatment phase; 92 vs. 67 percent, $p<.001$ over a two-year, follow-up period). Time to any recurrence was significantly longer for those in the psychoeducation group (log $rank_1 = 13.45$, $p<.001$). At the end of the 24-month, follow-up period, number of days of hospitalization was significantly more for those in the control group (14.83 vs. 4.75 days for those in psychoeducation, $p<.05$). Other research indicates that psychoeducation focusing on early recognition of manic symptoms is superior to routine care, with longer time periods before manic relapses and improved social-occupational functioning.[172] Educational programs can increase patient satisfaction with treatment and treatment compliance as well.[173, 174]

What is Family-Focused Treatment (FFT) for Bipolar Disorder?

FFT is a psychoeducational treatment approach that assumes that the environmental setting within which a patient resides is an important determinant of relapse likelihood. Therefore, family psychoeducation is administered once a patient has begun to stabilize from an acute episode. The program's goals are to educate patients and family members about the nature, symptoms, course, and treatment of bipolar illness, making it easier for them to deal with the disorder. Additionally, a focus on communication and problem-solving skills may reduce tension in the family environment.

FFT has been the subject of several controlled trials and is consequently the most well-known and validated family-based intervention for bipolar disorder.

FFT Treatment Strategies

FFT consists of 21 outpatient sessions held over nine months, administered concurrently with ongoing pharmacotherapy. At least one significant other (e.g., parent, spouse, sibling, supportive friend, caregiver) participates with the patient.

Generally, FFT includes three stages of treatment:[175]

1. **Family Psychoeducation** — This stage includes reviewing educational materials on the illness, symptoms, risk factors, and protective factors, origin of the disorder, medical and psychosocial treatments, and self-management. Clinicians present the biological and genetic underpinnings of bipolar disorder from a vulnerability-stress perspective that emphasizes that, for a person who has a genetic propensity to the disorder, environmental stress can bring on the disorder and affect symptom severity. They also emphasize the importance of treatment compliance. Additionally, this stage includes education about relapse prevention, in which participants work together to identify early warning signs and develop plans to prevent recurrence.

2. **Communication Enhancement Training** — In this stage, participants learn communication skills for dealing with family stress. These communication skills involve:

   ▶ *Active listening* — This training teaches participants to listen attentively and incorporate verbal meaning, underlying feelings, emotions, and body language to their understanding of communication. Active listening can include paraphrasing, or rephrasing someone's communication to ensure correct understanding. For example, the person may say, "I want to be sure I understand what you have said. You would like me to check with you before making purchases of more than $100. Is that correct?"

   ▶ **Expressing both positive and negative feelings** — For example, many people express their negative feelings, but neglect to mention those times when the behavior of another contributed to positive feelings. Communication enhancement training would emphasize relaying those messages, such as, "I felt very loved when you let me sleep late this morning."

   ▶ **Requesting adaptive changes in each other's behavior** — This training helps participants learn to request changes in their loved ones, without using attacking or accusing language. For example, instead of saying, "You never help me around the house, and you just think I am lazy," a better way of requesting a change might be, "I've been feeling more depressed and have less energy right now. I'd like to split up some household chores so that they aren't as overwhelming to me during this hard time."

These critical communication and assertion skills are taught through *behavioral rehearsal* and *role-playing*.

active listening — a way of listening that focuses entirely on what the other person is saying and confirms understanding of both the message content and the emotions and feelings underlying the message to ensure accurate understanding

behavioral rehearsal — rehearsing new responses to problematic situations

role-playing — helping their friend or family member acquire new communication skills by having them act out conversations in session

3. **Problem-solving Skills Training** — This final stage of FFT involves training participants to identify, define, and solve specific family problems related to bipolar disorder. For example, the family may be experiencing additional stress due to the patient having stopped working. This intervention may involve strategizing ways to cope with the reduced family income, staying within a budget, or discussing potential part- or full-time work options that may be feasible for the patient.

The FFT structure includes between-session homework so that patients and their loved ones can practice new skills in the home. For example, they may be asked to use new *assertive communication techniques* in conversation and then report back on their success and problems implementing the techniques in real-life applications.

Effectiveness of FFT

A number of studies have been conducted in recent years on the efficacy of FFT as an adjunct to medication therapy compared to:

- ▶ **Medication therapy alone** — FFT in addition to medication produced significantly less relapse (11 percent) than medication alone (61 percent) over a nine-month, follow-up period.[175]

- ▶ **Two family education sessions and follow-up crisis management** — In the first randomized comparison of these treatments (n=70) for patients receiving FFT, only 29 percent experienced a relapse into depression, compared to 53 percent in the family education/crisis management comparison treatment over a one-year, follow-up period.[176] A larger trial (n=101) indicated that patients receiving FFT compared to crisis management (two sessions of family education plus crisis intervention sessions as needed) experienced a 35 percent relapse rate, greater reduction in mood symptoms, and better medication adherence, compared to a 54 percent relapse rate, less reduction in mood symptoms, and poorer medication compliance for patients receiving crisis management.[177] Additionally, those in FFT averaged 73.5 weeks before a new mood episode versus 53.2 weeks for those in crisis management. Patients in both groups received concurrent medication treatment.

- ▶ **Individually-focused treatment** — Patients participating in a nine-month study of FFT (concurrent with medication treatment) had only a 28 percent relapse rate during a one-year, follow-up period. Comparatively, patients in the control group receiving individual supportive, problem-focused, and educational interventions

assertive communication techniques — these techniques help patients honestly express opinions, feelings, attitudes, and rights (without undue anxiety) in a way that doesn't infringe on the rights of others

(concurrent with medication treatment) experienced a 60 percent relapse rate over the same follow-up period. Additionally, only 12 percent of patients in FFT were hospitalized during the one-year, follow up period, compared to 60 percent in individually based treatment.[178]

What Individual Psychosocial Therapy Approaches are used to Treat Bipolar Disorder?

This section presents treatment strategies and efficacy research results for cognitive behavioral therapy (CBT) and interpersonal social rhythm therapy (IPSRT).

CBT theory can be related to the philosophy of the ancient Greeks, "Nothing in life is actually bad, lest we perceive it to be so."

CBT Treatment Strategies

Cognitive-behavioral therapy (CBT) is most often associated with the work of Albert Ellis and Aaron Beck, dating back to the early 1970s. The basic premise of this therapy is based on the theory that dysfunctional or chronic, intense emotions stem from distorted and irrational thoughts. These thoughts are internalized by the patient but impact their behaviors and patterns of social reinforcement. Thus, for CBT theorists, individuals' perceptions of life events can produce independent emotional and behavioral problems and potentially exacerbate symptoms of bipolar disorder and impact treatment response.

ACTIVATING EVENTS
(Situational Triggers)

BELIEFS
(Distorted and Irrational Thoughts)

=

CONSEQUENCES
(Depression, Anger, Suicide Attempts)

According to CBT, **"activating events"** (situational triggers) lead to **beliefs** (distorted and irrational thoughts), which lead to emotional and behavioral **consequences** (depression, anger, suicide attempts).

For example, being turned down for a date (an activating event) may trigger the person with bipolar disorder to have irrational thoughts (beliefs), such as:

- ▶ "He hates me," (rather than, "He said no to going on a date.")
- ▶ "Nobody will ever like me," (rather than, "Maybe I'm not his type.")
- ▶ "I'll never find anybody that will love me," (rather than, "The timing wasn't good for him; maybe he's involved with someone else.")
- ▶ "That's it! Trying to make new relationships will never work. I'll have to be alone for the rest of my life," (rather than, "Maybe next time, I'll find out more about the person as a friend, then I'll know more about whether or not to ask him out.")

The results of these thought processes could be behaviors (consequences), such as withdrawing from social interaction, becoming depressed, or perhaps attempting suicide.

The cognitive-behavioral approach to the treatment of bipolar disorder is based on two underlying assumptions:

1. Thoughts, feelings, and behaviors are interrelated.
2. Patients who are well educated about their illness are better prepared to participate in their treatment and recovery.

CBT is an active therapy that involves ongoing interaction between clinician and patient. Most often, it involves mutually agreed-upon goals for change, and continuously monitoring progress toward achieving those goals. For example, a patient and clinician may agree that minimizing irritable outbursts toward family members is a goal, and the patient will then keep a diary tracking unpleasant or hostile interactions with family members. It often includes homework assignments between sessions, such as completing relaxation exercises or practicing assertive communication skills. The goal of CBT is that the patient will learn new skills and strategies that they will eventually implement independently as needed.

While CBT is commonly used for a multitude of psychological problems and psychiatric disorders, the focus for patients with bipolar disorder is somewhat more specific. As summarized in Basco and Rush (1996), goals of CBT for patients with bipolar disorder include teaching patients (and often significant others):[179]

▶ About the disorder, treatment options, and common difficulties associated with the illness.

▶ Ways to monitor occurrence, severity, and course of manic and depressive symptoms and to change behaviors as needed (e.g., excessive daytime sleeping or gambling) and use structured problem solving as an alternative.

▶ Strategies for adhering to prescribed medication.

▶ How to use non-pharmacological strategies, specifically cognitive-behavioral skills, for coping with the cognitive, affective, and behavioral problems associated with manic and depressive symptoms. For example, the goal may be to reduce dysfunctional cognitions and emotions associated with symptoms that lead to maladaptive behavior (e.g., thoughts of worthlessness leading to suicidal behavior).

▶ Coping strategies for stressors that may interfere with treatment or precipitate episodes of mania and/or depression.

The psychosocial modalities for treating bipolar disorder have substantial overlap.

Although many CBT-based theoretical interventions include some elements of psychoeducation, they also include cognitive restructuring and behavioral approaches, which differentiate them from a strictly psychoeducational approach to treatment.

As discussed in the section on psychoeducational interventions, education may be multifaceted, and could include ongoing symptom monitoring for early detection and interventions for emergent mood symptoms, coping with symptoms and consequences of bipolar disorder, and improving psychosocial problem management.

Effectiveness of CBT

Several studies indicate that CBT is a helpful adjunct to pharmacotherapy for persons with bipolar disorder. One such study examined the effects of medication plus a six-session CBT protocol focusing on medication adherence (for lithium treatment).[175] The combined treatment group demonstrated significantly better compliance with lithium and fewer hospitalizations over a six-month, follow-up period than the lithium-only group. The study used global medical regimen adherence measures, including patient reports, physicians' ratings, chart notations, and serum lithium blood levels.

A more recent study examined the effects of teaching patients to recognize emergent episode symptoms and then rehearsing an action plan for seeking care, thus demonstrating the significant educational component of CBT. For example, the CBT intervention assisted patients in recognizing early mood symptoms and then generating strategies (such as seeing their doctor) for immediate interventions to prevent further symptom acceleration. In this study, which compared CBT to routine care, the intervention was associated with 30 percent fewer manic relapses, greater time to manic relapse, and significantly better social functioning over an 18-month, follow-up period. However, CBT was ineffective in reducing depressive relapses.[172]

A 2001 study randomized 42 patients with bipolar disorder to either CBT or a treatment-as-usual, waiting-list condition (no psychosocial therapy) in addition to routine medication management. In this study, the CBT consisted of psychoeducation and specific discussion of the importance and tactics to optimize medication adherence, stress management, cognitive restructuring, and regulation of activities and sleep.[181]

At the six-month follow-up, patients who received CBT achieved statistically significant reductions in:

Global Assessment of Function (GAF) Score — score from 0–100 that indicates the patient's level of functioning

- ▶ **Global Assessment of Function (GAF) score** — The CBT group increased an average of 16.4 points vs. only 3.9 points for the control group (p<.05).

- ▶ **Depressive symptoms** (using the Beck Depression Inventory) — The CBT group's scores decreased by 7.3 points vs. the control group's scores that increased by 2.5 points (p<.02). Furthermore, a follow-up of 29 control patients, who were switched to the CBT treatment group (after being on the waiting list for six months), indicated a 60 percent reduction in relapse over the 18 months after the switch than those who remained in the control group.[181]

A 2003 study randomized 103 patients with bipolar I disorder to receive either cognitive therapy (CT group) or serve in a control condition.[182] Both groups received minimal psychiatric care, defined as mood stabilizers at a recommended level and routine psychiatric follow-up.

The CT group received an average of 14 sessions of cognitive therapy during the first six months and two booster sessions in the final six months of the study, with a focus on reducing depression symptoms as well as preventing new mood episodes.

Results indicate that those in the CT group experienced significantly fewer bipolar episodes and mood symptoms over the 12-month period. Medication compliance was rated by physicians as higher for patients in the CT group, and there appeared to be a benefit in promoting social functioning as well.

IPSRT Strategies

Interpersonal Social Rhythm Therapy (IPSRT) is a short-term and present-focused, individual therapy derived from the interpersonal psychosocial therapy used to treat depression.[183, 184] The philosophy of traditional interpersonal therapy is that, for individuals genetically prone to bipolar disorder, stressful interpersonal events may contribute to the onset of symptoms, **particularly depressive symptoms**. Thus, this approach focuses on the interpersonal context in which depression symptoms emerge. Patients learn to identify problematic social patterns and relate their moods to these patterns.

Clinicians help patients determine which of the following core problem areas may be contributing to their symptoms:

▶ Grief over loss (including "grieving the lost healthy self")

▶ Interpersonal conflicts

▶ Role transitions

▶ Interpersonal skills deficits

The patient then learns ways to resolve current problems and hopefully prevent their reemergence.

Grief over Loss (including "grieving the lost healthy self")

The clinician assesses for the presence of *abnormal grief*. In some cases, this form of grief includes grieving over the lost "healthy" self or opportunities missed due to illness. For example, a person may grieve the fact that they never finished college, as they became incapacitated by symptoms during that time of their life and dropped out. Abnormal grief can also include delayed grief responses, in which a person grieves long after the loss. For example, the patient who has recently turned 42 may experience new and profound grief over the death of her own mother, who died at the same age 20 years previously.

Although an IPSRT-based theoretical intervention packages some elements of psychoeducation, it focuses on interpersonal contexts in which symptoms (particularly depression symptoms) emerge, helping patients identify problematic social patterns and relate their moods to these patterns. This focus is what differentiates IPSRT from a strictly psychoeducational approach to treatment.

abnormal grief — acute grief persisting beyond the typical two to four months that may contribute to depressive symptoms or exacerbate a bipolar depressive episode

Depression treatment goals associated with grief center on facilitating the mourning process and helping the patient re-establish interests and relationships that can substitute for what has been lost.

Interpersonal Conflicts

The patient and a significant other may have ongoing conflicting expectations about their relationship that may contribute to symptoms. Treatment goals include identifying the disputes, making choices about a plan of action, and then modifying communication patterns and/or reassessing expectations to resolve the dispute. For example, an unemployed person with bipolar disorder may have accumulated significant debt from previous spending sprees while symptomatic and expect family members to resolve those debts for them. This results in ongoing conflict and arguments with family members. In this situation, the patient may work with the clinician to improve communication and persuasion skills, so that they can discuss their expectations and needs with their family in a reasonable and successful way. Alternatively, the patient may revise expectations, and begin to work toward resolving their financial problems through other means.

Role Transitions (changes in one's job or family situation)

When a person has difficulty coping with life changes that require a role change, the clinician will work with the patient to give up a previous role; express anger, guilt, or loss; acquire new skills; and develop new attachments and support groups. For example, a person may experience a divorce, and have mood symptoms as a consequence of their dissatisfaction with life events and their new status as a single person. The clinician and patient may work together to recognize the positive aspects of single life and the dissolution of an unhappy marriage, enhance the person's social contacts, and acclimate to this role change.

Interpersonal Skill Deficits
(e.g., poor conversational skills, dependence)

Those with long histories of inadequate or superficial interpersonal relationships may have deficits that lead to social isolation.

The interpersonal therapy model predicts that interpersonal deficits can contribute to mood symptoms. This area of treatment seeks to reduce social isolation and help the patient acquire skills to build more intimate and lasting relationships. The clinician may help the patient identify the characteristics of previously successful relationships, such as those built around shared interests (e.g., woodworking, pottery, travel). The clinician may then suggest enrolling in a related class or joining a special interest group to improve the patient's social interactions.

Unique for bipolar disorder, IPSRT focuses overall on the role of stressful life events on a patient's social and circadian rhythms. The underlying premise is that symptoms result from changes in sleep routines, changes in social stimulation, and neurotransmitter dysregulation. Patients learn to monitor the interrelations between their daily routines, sleep, levels of social stimulation, and mood as well as how a change in one domain affects others.

For example, a patient may recognize that they tend to experience emergent hypomanic symptoms when they sleep irregularly, or less than eight hours per night. When generating possible solutions to that pattern, the patient may consider using prescribed medications, a warm bath at bedtime, or other interventions to ensure getting eight hours of sleep each night.

In later phases of treatment, patients work toward regulating their daily routines and sleep/wake cycles and finding optimal balances among these factors. They also learn to anticipate and develop plans for coping with events that might be disruptive to established routines. For example, a shift worker may work with the clinician to cope with the supervisor's occasional requests that he work a double shift that could potentially disrupt his sleep-wake routine. They may rehearse an appropriate response to that request, respectfully declining the extra hours.

Effectiveness of IPSRT

A large maintenance trial, based at the University of Pittsburgh, is currently studying the effectiveness of IPSRT in addition to medication therapy versus intensive clinical management (ICM) as an adjunctive treatment. ICM group participants also attend one-on-one sessions with a clinician, but the content of those meetings is limited to discussion of symptoms, education, medication adherence, and management of side effects. Study authors describe ICM as "low-dose" psychosocial therapy, compared to the more intensive, "high-dose" psychosocial intervention of IPSRT.[162, 185]

The study requires 12 weeks of preliminary treatment, during which time patients receive pharmacotherapy and attend sessions with a clinician, randomized to either IPSRT or ICM. Preliminary analyses on the first 38 participants suggested IPSRT is effective in increasing the stability of daily routines and sleep/wake cycles, as measured by their Social Rhythm Metric Scores.[185] Those patients who completed at least one year of IPSRT were more likely to maintain euthymic states and less likely to develop depressive states than patients in ICM.[186, 187]

Further analyses of this trial (n=82) suggested that patients who received the same treatment modality throughout their participation (either ICM exclusively or IPSRT exclusively, versus some of each), had lower rates of recurrence (20 vs 40 percent) over the 52-week, follow-up period.

Adding psychosocial interventions to pharmacological treatments may optimize bipolar disorder treatment by:

▶ Substantially improving medication adherence

▶ Enhancing clinical and functional outcomes

These interventions are individually tailored to the needs of the specific patient, but are designed to protect and preserve essential social rhythms and routines. For example, when attending a family reunion with many people, high levels of social stimulation, and changes in routine and schedule, the person with bipolar disorder may reserve a room in a nearby hotel, to allow time away from the intense social atmosphere for rest and renewal.

In addition, IPSRT may help promote euthymic periods for those with bipolar disorder.[185]

These findings only include a small number of patients, and the results of the larger trial will provide more insight and information about the use and effectiveness of this approach.

> ► Reducing symptoms
> ► Increasing periods of wellness between mood episodes

As with all interventions, the choice to add psychosocial interventions should be carefully weighed through conversation between care provider and patient, considering both the potential positive effects as well as possible risks. A recent review of psychoeducation and CBT highlighted two such risks:[154]

1. Greater awareness of depressive symptoms and early symptom detection has been linked with increased antidepressant use, with no associated reduction in episodes.[172] Therefore, education should also include instruction in alternate coping strategies for depressive symptoms.

2. Having greater knowledge of the disorder has been associated with increased anxiety during the early phases of treatment.[188] This can be alleviated by providing appropriate support.

Further research is needed on the mechanisms of psychosocial interventions, including what aspects are most important to obtain positive results, to further understand how to best combine treatments for individuals with bipolar disorder.

Key Concepts for Chapter Four:

1. Research demonstrates that psychosocial interventions are helpful adjuncts to traditional pharmacological treatment of bipolar disorder. They appear to reduce acute symptoms, prevent new episodes, increase compliance with medication, and decrease rates of hospitalization.

2. Psychosocial interventions can help teach patients strategies to improve coping with stressful life events, increase social support networks, regularize sleep-wake cycles, and identify and control psychological mechanisms that may exacerbate bipolar illness.

3. Most psychosocial interventions are diverse, and employ a variety of techniques and interventions based on the unique needs of an individual.

4. Most psychosocial treatment packages include some form of psychoeducation (teaching the patient and/or family members about the illness, treatments, and relapse prevention).

5. Therapies with research evidence to support their effectiveness for patients with bipolar disorder include family-focused therapy (FFT), cognitive-behavioral therapies (CBT), and interpersonal social rhythm therapy (IPSRT).

Appendix A:
DSM-IV (TR) Diagnostic Criteria

Criteria for Major Depressive Episode

A. Five (or more) of the following symptoms have been present during the same 2-week period and represent a change from previous functioning; at least one of the symptoms is either (1) depressed mood or (2) loss of interest or pleasure.

Note: Do not include symptoms that are clearly due to a general medical condition, or mood-incongruent delusions or hallucinations.

(1) depressed mood most of the day, nearly every day, as indicated by either subjective report (e.g., feels sad or empty) or observation made by others (e.g., appears tearful). **Note:** In children and adolescents, can be irritable mood.

(2) markedly diminished interest or pleasure in all, or almost all, activities most of the day, nearly every day (as indicated by either subjective account or observation made by others)

(3) significant weight loss when not dieting or weight gain (e.g., a change of more than 5% of body weight in a month), or decrease or increase in appetite nearly every day. **Note:** In children, consider failure to make expected weight gains.

(4) insomnia or hypersomnia nearly every day

(5) psychomotor agitation or retardation nearly every day (observable by others, not merely subjective feelings of restlessness or being slowed down)

(6) fatigue or loss of energy nearly every day

(7) feelings of worthlessness or excessive or inappropriate guilt (which may be delusional) nearly every day (not merely self-reproach or guilt about being sick)

(8) diminished ability to think or concentrate, or indecisiveness, nearly ever day (either by subjective account or as observed by others)

(9) recurrent thoughts of death (not just fear of dying), recurrent suicidal ideation without a specific plan, or a suicide attempt or a specific plan for committing suicide

B. The symptoms do not meet criteria for a Mixed Episode.

This appendix presents diagnostic criteria relevant for bipolar disorder assessment, reprinted with permission from the American Psychological Association, as follows:

► *Criteria for Major Depressive Episode*

► *Criteria for Manic Episode*

► *Criteria for Mixed Episode*

► *Criteria for Hypomanic Episode*

► *Diagnostic criteria for 296.0x Bipolar I Disorder, Single Manic Episode*

► *Diagnostic Criteria for 296.40 Bipolar I Disorder, Most Recent Episode Hypomanic*

► *Diagnostic criteria for 296.4x Bipolar I Disorder, Most Recent Episode Manic*

► *Diagnostic criteria for 296.5x Bipolar I Disorder, Most Recent Episode Depressed*

► *Diagnostic criteria for 296.6x Bipolar I Disorder, Most Recent Episode Mixed*

► *Diagnostic criteria for 296.7 Bipolar I Disorder, Most Recent Episode Unspecified*

► *Diagnostic criteria for 296.89 Bipolar II Disorder*

► *Diagnostic criteria for 301.13 Cyclothymic Disorder*

C. The symptoms cause clinically significant distress or impairment in social, occupational or other important areas of functioning.

D. The symptoms are not due to the direct physiological effects of a substance (e.g., a drug of abuse, a medication) or a general medical condition (e.g., hypothyroidism).

E. The symptoms are not better accounted for by Bereavement, i.e., after the loss of a loved one, the symptoms persist for longer than 2 months or are characterized by marked functional impairment, morbid preoccupation with worthlessness, suicidal ideation, psychotic symptoms, or psychomotor retardation.

Criteria for Manic Episode

A. A distinct period of abnormally and persistently elevated, expansive, or irritable mood, lasting at least 1 week (or any duration if hospitalization is necessary).

B. During the period of mood disturbance, three (or more) of the following symptoms have persisted (four if the mood is only irritable) and have been present to a significant degree:

    (1)   Inflated self-esteem or grandiosity

    (2)   Decreased need for sleep (e.g., feels rested after only 3 hours of sleep)

    (3)   More talkative than usual or pressure to keep talking

    (4)   Flight of ideas or subjective experience that thoughts are racing

    (5)   Distractibility (i.e., attention too easily drawn to unimportant or irrelevant external stimuli)

    (6)   Increase in goal-directed activity (either socially, at work or school, or sexually) or psychomotor agitation

    (7)   Excessive involvement in pleasurable activities that have a high potential for painful consequences (e.g., engaging in unrestrained buying sprees, sexual indiscretions, or foolish investments)

C. The symptoms do not meet criteria for a Mixed Episode.

D. The mood disturbance is sufficiently severe to cause marked impairment in occupational functioning or in usual social activities or relationships with others, or to necessitate hospitalization to prevent harm to self or others, or there are psychotic features.

E. The symptoms are not due to the direct physiological effects of a substance (e.g., a drug of abuse, a medication, or other treatment) or a general medical condition (e.g., hyperthyroidism). **Note:** Manic-like episodes that are clearly caused by somatic antidepressant treatment (e.g., medication, electroconvulsive therapy, light therapy) should not count toward a diagnosis of Bipolar I Disorder.

Criteria for Mixed Episode

A. The criteria are met both for a Manic Episode and for a Major Depressive Episode (except for duration) nearly every day during at least a 1-week period.

B. The mood disturbance is sufficiently severe to cause marked impairment in occupational functioning or in usual social activities or relationships with others, or to neces- sitate hospitalization to prevent harm to self or others, or there are psychotic features.

C. The symptoms are not due to the direct physiological effects of a substance (e.g., a drug of abuse, a medication, or other treatment) or a general medical condition (e.g., hyperthyroidism).

Note: Mixed-like episodes that are clearly caused by somatic antidepressant treatment (e.g., medication, electroconvulsive therapy, light therapy) should not count toward a diagnosis of Bipolar I Disorder.

Criteria for Hypomanic Episode

A. A distinct period of persistently elevated, expansive, or irri- table mood, lasting throughout at least 4 days, that is clearly different from the usual nondepressed mood.

B. During the period of mood disturbance, three (or more) of the following symptoms have persisted (four if the mood is only irritable) and have been present to a significant degree:

(1) Inflated self-esteem or grandiosity

(2) Decreased need for sleep (e.g., feels rested after only 3 hours of sleep)

(3) More talkative than usual or pressure to keep talking

(4) Flight of ideas or subjective experience that thoughts are racing

(5) Distractibility (i.e., attention too easily drawn to unim- portant or irrelevant external stimuli)

(6) Increase in goal-directed activity (either socially, at work or school, or sexually) or psychomotor agitation

(7) Excessive involvement in pleasurable activities that have a high potential for painful consequences (e.g., the person engages in unrestrained buying sprees, sexual indiscretions, or foolish business investments)

C. The episode is associated with an unequivocal change in functioning that is uncharacteristic of the person when not symptomatic.

D. The disturbance in mood and the change in functioning are observable by others.

E. The episode is not severe enough to cause marked impairment in social or occupational functioning, or to necessitate hospitalization, and there are no psychotic features.

F. The symptoms are not due to the direct physiological effects of a substance (e.g., a drug of abuse, a medication, or other treatment) or a general medical condition (e.g., hyperthyroidism). **Note:** Hypomanic-like episodes that are clearly caused by somatic antidepressant treatment (e.g., medication, electroconvulsive therapy, light therapy) should not count toward a diagnosis of Bipolar II Disorder.

Diagnostic criteria for 296.0x Bipolar I Disorder, Single Manic Episode

A. Presence of only one Manic Episode and no past Major Depressive Episodes. **Note:** Recurrence is defined as either a change in polarity from depression or an interval of at least 2 months without manic symptoms.

B. The Manic Episode is not better accounted for by Schizoaffective Disorder and is not superimposed on Schizophrenia, Schizophreniform Disorder, Delusional Disorder, or Psychotic Disorder Not Otherwise Specified.

Specify if:

Mixed: if symptoms meet criteria for a Mixed Episode

If the full criteria are currently met for a Manic, Mixed, or Major Depressive Episode, specify its current clinical status and/or features:

Mild, Moderate, Severe Without Psychotic Features/Severe With Psychotic Features

With Catatonic Features
With Postpartum Onset

If the full criteria are not currently met for a Manic, Mixed, or Major Depressive Episode, specify the current clinical status of the Bipolar I Disorder or features of the most recent episode:
In Partial Remission, In Full Remission

With Catatonic Features

With Postpartum Onset

Diagnostic Criteria for 296.40 Bipolar I Disorder, Most Recent Episode Hypomanic

A. Currently (or most recently) in a Hypomanic Episode

B. There has previously been at least one Manic Episode or Mixed Episode.

C. The mood symptoms cause clinically significant distress or impairment in social, occupational, or other important areas of functioning.

D. The mood episodes in Criteria A and B are not better accounted for by Schizoaffective Disorder and are not superimposed on Schizophrenia, Schizophreniform Disorder, Delusional Disorder, or Psychotic Disorder Not Otherwise Specified.

Specify:

Longitudinal Course Specifiers (With and Without Interepisode Recovery)

With Seasonal Pattern (applies only to the pattern of Major Depressive Episodes)

With Rapid Cycling

Diagnostic criteria for 296.4x Bipolar I Disorder, Most Recent Episode Manic

A. Currently (or most recently) in a Manic Episode

B. There has previously been at least one Major Depressive Episode, Manic Episode, or Mixed Episode.

C. The mood episodes in Criteria A and B are not better accounted for by Schizoaffective Disorder and are not superimposed on Schizophrenia, Schizophreniform Disorder, Delusional Disorder, or Psychotic Disorder Not Otherwise Specified.

If the full criteria are currently met for a Manic Episode, specify its current clinical status and/or features:

Mild, Moderate, Severe Without Psychotic Features/Severe With Psychotic Features

With Catatonic Features

With Postpartum Onset

If the full criteria are not currently met for a Manic Episode, specify its current clinical status of the Bipolar I Disorder and/or features of the most recent Manic Episode:

In Partial Remission, In Full Remission

With Catatonic Features

With Postpartum Onset

Specify:

> Longitudinal Course Specifiers (With and Without Interepisode Recovery)
>
> With Seasonal Pattern (applies only to the pattern of Major Depressive Episodes)
>
> With Rapid Cycling

Diagnostic criteria for 296.6x Bipolar I Disorder, Most Recent Episode Mixed

A. Currently (or most recently) in a Mixed Episode

B. There has previously been at least one Major Depressive Episode, Manic Episode, or Mixed Episode.

C. The mood episodes in Criteria A and B are not better accounted for by Schizoaffective Disorder and are not superimposed on Schizophrenia, Schizophreniform Disorder, Delusional Disorder, or Psychotic Disorder Not Otherwise Specified.

If the full criteria are currently met for a Mixed Episode, specify its current clinical status and/or features:

> Mild, Moderate, Severe Without Psychotic Features/Severe With Psychotic Features
>
> With Catatonic Features
>
> With Postpartum Onset

If the full criteria are not currently met for a Mixed Episode, specify its current clinical status of the Bipolar I Disorder and/or features of the most recent Mixed Episode:

> In Partial Remission, In Full Remission
>
> With Catatonic Features
>
> With Postpartum Onset

Specify:

> Longitudinal Course Specifiers (With and Without Interepisode Recovery)
>
> With Seasonal Pattern (applies only to the pattern of Major Depressive Episodes)
>
> With Rapid Cycling

Diagnostic criteria for 296.5x Bipolar I Disorder, Most Recent Episode Depressed

A. Currently (or most recently) in a Major Depressive Episode

B. There has previously been at least one Manic Episode, Mixed Episode

C. The mood episodes in Criteria A and B are not better accounted for by Schizoaffective Disorder and are not superimposed on Schizophrenia, Schizophreniform Disorder, Delusional Disorder, or Psychotic Disorder Not Otherwise Specified.

If the full criteria are currently met for a Major Depressive Episode, specify its current clinical status and/or features:

> Mild, Moderate, Severe Without Psychotic Features/Severe With Psychotic Features
>
> Chronic
>
> With Catatonic Features
>
> With Melancholic Features
>
> With Atypical Features
>
> With Postpartum Onset

If the full criteria are currently met for a Major Depressive Episode, specify the current clinical status of the Bipolar I Disorder and/or features of the most recent Major Depressive Episode:

> In Partial Remission, In Full Remission
>
> Chronic
>
> With Catatonic Features
>
> With Melancholic Features
>
> With Atypical Features
>
> With Postpartum Onset

Specify:

> Longitudinal Course Specifiers (With and Without Interepisode Recovery)
>
> With Seasonal Pattern (applies only to the pattern of Major Depressive Episodes)
>
> With Rapid Cycling

Diagnostic criteria for 296.7 Bipolar I Disorder, Most Recent Episode Unspecified

A. Criteria, except for duration, are currently (or most recently) met for a Manic, a Hypomanic, a Mixed, or a Major Depressive Episode

B. There has previously been at least one Manic Episode or Mixed Episode.

C. The mood symptoms cause clinically significant distress or impairment in social, occupational, or other important areas of functioning.

D. The mood symptoms in Criteria A and B are not better accounted for by Schizoaffective Disorder and are not superimposed on Schizophrenia, Schizophreniform Disorder, Delusional Disorder, or Psychotic Disorder Not Otherwise Specified.

E. The mood symptoms in Criteria A and B are not due to the direct physiological effects of a substance (e.g., a drug of abuse, a medication, or other treatment) or a general medical condition (e.g., hyperthyroidism).

Specify:

  Longitudinal Course Specifiers (With and Without Interepisode Recovery)

  With Seasonal Pattern (applies only to the pattern of Major Depressive Episodes)

  With Rapid Cycling

Diagnostic criteria for 296.89 Bipolar II Disorder

A. Presence (or history) of one or more Major Depressive Episodes

B. Presence (or history) of at least one Hypomanic Episode

C. There has never been a Manic Episode or a Mixed Episode

D. The mood symptoms in Criteria A and B are not better accounted for by Schizoaffective Disorder and are not superimposed on Schizophrenia, Schizophreniform Disorder, Delusional Disorder, or Psychotic Disorder Not Otherwise Specified.

E. The symptoms cause clinically significant distress or impairment in social, occupational, or other important areas of functioning.

Specify current or most recent episode:

  Hypomanic: if currently (or most recently) in a Hypomanic Episode

  Depressed: if currently (or most recently) in a Major Depressive Episode

If the full criteria are currently met for a Major Depressive Episode, specify its current clinical status and/or features:

Mild, Moderate, Severe Without Psychotic Features/Severe With Psychotic Features

Note: Fifth-digit codes specified cannot be used here because the code for Bipolar II Disorder already uses the fifth digit.

Chronic

With Catatonic Features

With Melancholic Features

With Atypical Features

With Postpartum Onset

If the full criteria are currently met for a Hypomanic or Major Depressive Episode, specify its clinical status of the Bipolar II Disorder and/or features of the most recent Major Depressive Episode (only if it is the most recent type of mood episode):

In Partial Remission, In Full Remission

Note: Fifth-digit codes specified cannot be used here because the code for Bipolar II Disorder already uses the fifth digit.

Chronic

With Catatonic Features

With Melancholic Features

With Atypical Features

With Postpartum Onset

Specify:

Longitudinal Course Specifiers (With and Without Interepisode Recovery)

With Seasonal Pattern (applies only to the pattern of Major Depressive Episodes)

With Rapid Cycling

Diagnostic criteria for 301.13 Cyclothymic Disorder

A. For at least 2 years, the presence of numerous periods with hypomanic symptoms and numerous periods with depressive symptoms that do not meet criteria for a Major Depressive Episode.

Note: In children and adolescents, the duration must be at least 1 year.

B. During the above 2-year period (1 year in children and adolescents), the person has not been without the symptoms in Criterion A for more than 2 months at a time.

C. No Major Depressive Episode, Manic Episode, or Mixed Episode has been present during the first 2 years of the disturbance.

Note: After the initial 2 years (1 year in children and adolescents) of Cyclothymic Disorder, there may be superimposed Manic or Mixed Episodes (in which case both Bipolar I Disorder and Cyclothymic Disorder may be diagnosed) or Major Depressive Episodes (in which case both Bipolar II Disorder and Cyclothymic Disorder may be diagnosed).

D. The symptoms in Criteria A are not better accounted for by Schizoaffective Disorder and are not superimposed on Schizophrenia, Schizophreniform Disorder, Delusional Disorder, or Psychotic Disorder Not Otherwise Specified.

E. The symptoms are not due to the direct physiological effects of a substance (e.g., a drug of abuse, a medication) or a general medical condition (e.g., hyperthyroidism).

F. The symptoms cause clinically significant distress or impairment in social, occupational, or other important areas of functioning.

Appendix B:
Structured Tools for Assessing Bipolar Disorder

Using Structured Clinical Interviews

CLINICAL interviewing tools for diagnosing bipolar disorder include:

▶ The Schedule for Affective Disorders and Schizophrenia (SADS)
▶ Diagnostic Interview Schedule (DIS)
▶ The Structured Clinical Interview for the DSM-IV (SCID)

SADS

Developed to differentiate between affective disorders and schizophrenia, the SADS must be administered by trained professionals. It is designed to evaluate current and lifetime affective disorders and yields diagnoses consistent with research criteria for bipolar disorder, depression, and other diagnostic categories.

The instrument is a semi-structured interview divided into two parts and takes approximately 1.5 to 2 hours to administer.

▶ Part I obtains a detailed description of the clinical features of the current episode and during the week prior to the interview.
▶ Part II obtains historical information needed to confirm a lifetime diagnosis. It also provides estimates of severity.

Questions are progressive and have built-in criteria for whether or not to rule out the symptoms for current diagnostic purposes.

Overall, the regular SADS has demonstrated excellent reliability, particularly for interrater and test-retest reliabilities related to current episodes of psychiatric disturbance.

DIS

The DIS is highly structured, diagnostic interview designed to be administered by experienced lay interviewers without clinical training.[37] The DIS has been used in psychiatric survey research for decades to assess the prevalence of psychiatric disorders in the general population. Modules cover mood, anxiety, schizophrenia, eating, *somatization,* psychoactive substance abuse, and antisocial personality disorders. The DIS provides both current and lifetime diagnostic information. Its content directly corresponds to DSM diagnostic criteria, and it has been updated periodically to correspond to the most current version [DSM-IV (TR)]. The computerized version can be self administered with availability of an assistant to answer questions if needed. Research supports the existence of compatible diagnoses by professionals and paraprofessionals using the DIS.[189]

somatization — multiple physical complaints involving any body system

81

Data on the reliability of diagnosis using the DIS, versus clinical judgment, is variable. This is expected, based upon the problems of relying on psychiatrist ratings as the "gold standard" of diagnosis. It has been suggested that these data be considered a form of interrater reliability, versus concurrent validity.

SCID

The SCID is a structured, broad-spectrum instrument that adheres closely to the DSM-IV decision trees for psychiatric diagnosis.[38] There are multiple versions, including a briefer clinical version, research version, and a module to assess for the presence of personality disorders. The SCID is designed for use by trained interviewers to ensure a structured and consistent format for investigating psychiatric symptoms.

The SCID and its variations include some open-ended questions and a skip pattern (i.e., negative responses to certain questions cause the interviewer to skip ahead in the instrument), which results in a shorter administration time for those with fewer symptoms. Trained professional interviewers administer the SCID, as clinical judgment is required throughout the interview.

Research on the reliability of the SCID has found variable test-retest and interrater reliabilities, varying by diagnostic categories. Validity studies of the SCID have assumed that DSM-based diagnostic categories are the benchmark for making comparisons of diagnostic accuracy. Thus, "procedural validity" is assumed, as the SCID closely mirrors the criteria specified in DSM versions.[190]

Using Clinician-Administered Observational Rating Scales

A number of assessment tools exist that involve a combination of structured to semi-structured interview and behavioral observations, designed for administration by a trained interviewer because:

 ▶ Interviewer bias can occur, in which an interviewer systematically rates in a certain direction (e.g., rating the patient as more severely ill to justify continued treatment).

 ▶ Differences in training and administration of the scale can impact the applicability of results.

 ▶ Variations in the interview environment (interviewer and patient mood, distractions, behavior, etc.) can alter results.

Those clinician-administered instruments **commonly used with manic symptoms** include the Young Mania Rating Scale (YMRS) and the Clinician Administered Rating Scale for Mania (CARS-M).

YMRS

This 11-item measure was designed to measure the severity of manic symptoms and to detect the effects of treatment on mania.[39] It includes both mild and severe versions of manic symptoms. Items are ranked on a scale of 0–4 or 0–8. Professionals can administer the YMRS after minimal training.

The YMRS has demonstrated good *interrater* and *interitem reliability,* and has a strong association to other measures of manic symptoms. It is typically utilized as the "gold standard" measurement of manic symptoms in research settings.

CARS-M

The CARS-M was designed to evaluate the severity of manic and psychotic symptoms, and to detect changes in such symptoms over the course of treatment.[40] It includes two subscales that are individually scored, measuring mania and psychosis respectively. Items assessing mania were derived from the SADS, described above. The scale includes 15 items that are rated from 0–6 on a Likert scale, except for one item, insight, which is rated 0–4. Each item has anchors, and the scale also includes prompts to aid clinicians in probing certain symptom domains. Clinicians are also permitted to use collateral information, such as family and medical histories, when making ratings.

Reliability for the CARS-M is substantial.[40] Additionally, the CARS-M correlates strongly (0.94) with the YMRS. Research evidence exists that the manic subscale can differentiate manic patients from those with other severe psychiatric disturbance.[40]

Those clinician-rated scales **commonly used to assess depressive symptoms** include the Hamilton Rating Scale for Depression (HAM-D), Montgomery-Äsberg Depression Rating Scale (MADRS), and the Inventory of Depressive Symptomatology-Clinician Rated (IDS-C).

HAM-D

Historically, the HAM-D is the most common interview method for assessing depression and was initially created to assess depression severity in those already diagnosed.[42-44] It has become a common outcome measure for evaluating the effects of different treatment interventions, especially drug therapies and inpatient treatments. The HAM-D is a 21-item scale completed during a 30-minute interview (only the first 17 items are scored, thus the scale is often referred to as the "HAM-17"). It includes a checklist of ranked on a scale of 0–4 or 0–2, and was designed to be administered by physicians, psychologists, and social workers, who have experience with psychiatric populations. However, the HAM-D can be administered by non-clinicians after some training.

interrater reliability — degree that different raters agree on a diagnosis based on the use of the instrument

interitem reliability — degree to which scores on individual items agree with each other; an estimate of the extent to which the instrument is measuring a single construct.

Both a computerized version and a paper-and-pencil, self-report version of the HAM-D are available.

The internal consistency is higher with use of the structured interview form.[191] Reports of interrater reliability have been consistent and high, ranging from 0.65–0.9 for the total score. Results from the HAM-D are highly correlated with results from other observer-rated instruments, such as the MADRS and IDS, and range from 0.80–0.90.

MADRS

The MADRS requires minimal training, and the authors state that professionals and nonprofessionals can administer the scale.

The MADRS is a clinician-rated measure, which provides data on overall depression severity and specific depressive symptoms.[45–47] It has been demonstrated to be sensitive to change in depression symptoms over time. The MADRS includes 10 items, which are rated on a scale of 0–6. Observations as well as verbal information are used in the ratings.

The reliability of the MADRS is acceptable and comparable to other observer-rated depression scales, with joint reliability for the total scale ranging from 0.76–0.95. The following mean scores from the MADRS correlate with global severity measures from the DSM: very severe, 44; severe, 31; moderate, 25; mild, 15; and recovered, 7.[46]

IDS-C

This measure was designed to capture symptoms of depression in both inpatients and outpatients, and is derived from diagnostic criteria for Major Depressive Disorder found in the DSM-IV.[41] It includes self-report and clinician-rated forms. It is unique in its efforts to be more comprehensive, including coverage of atypical and melancholic features as well as somatic and cognitive features of depression. The clinician-rated version includes 30 items, which are scored on a four-point anchored scale. It includes a semi-structured interview to assist a trained clinician interviewer.

The IDS-C possesses excellent reliability, achieving an internal consistency of 0.94 in a large sample. It is highly correlated with other depression rating scales.

Using Self-Ratings

Self-ratings are completed independently by the patient and help detect the presence or absence of symptoms. Three self-report instruments developed specifically for bipolar disorder are the Life Chart method, the Internal State Scale (ISS), and the Mood Disorder Questionnaire (MDQ).[48-51]

The Life Chart Method

This tool asks the patient to log daily specific information on their mood, sleep, medications, and life events. Copies of this daily log tool are in the public domain and available through the Depression Bipolar Support Alliance (DBSA) — www.dbsalliance.org. With clinician assistance, it can also be used to retrospectively retrace the course of illness.

Appendix C includes more information and a copy of the Life Chart instructions and sample log.

ISS

This tool is a 17-item, self report scale that includes assessment of both manic and depressive symptoms. Items are presented as a visual analog scale, respondents mark their response along the scale from 0 to 100. It can be useful in assessing mixed states as well as classic mania and depression. Factor analysis of the ISS reveals four subscales, called Activation, Perceived Conflict, Well-Being, and Depression. The ISS can be completed in approximately 15–20 minutes.

MDQ

The MDQ is a self-report diagnostic instrument, designed to be a brief, self-administered screening for bipolar disorder.[52] This tool serves as a brief diagnostic screening instrument for the presence of bipolar disorder, but provides little information about the severity and duration of symptoms.[52] It includes 13, "yes/no" items derived from both DSM-IV criteria and clinical experience. A positive screen requires that:

- ▶ Seven or more items must be endorsed.
- ▶ Several of the items must co-occur.
- ▶ The symptoms cause at least moderate psychosocial impairment.

The instrument demonstrated good *sensitivity* (0.73) and very good *specificity* (0.90) in outpatients treated at five outpatient psychiatric clinics. In contrast, when tested in a national epidemiological sample, the instrument correctly identified only 28.1 percent (weighted sensitivity) of those with SCID diagnoses of bipolar spectrum.[53] On the other hand, the MDQ identified 97.2 percent of the SCID individuals without bipolar disorder as "not bipolar" (weighted specificity). This scale may be a useful

sensitivity — the degree to which the instrument correctly identifies patients that **do have** the disorder

specificity — the degree to which the instrument correctly identifies patients that **do not have** the disorder

adjunct to other assessments because it is brief, and patients can complete it independently in the waiting room. However, diagnostic decisions cannot be made based on the MDQ alone.

Other Self-report Scales

Other scales used for assessing bipolar disorder include:

> ▶ **The Altman Mania Rating Scale (AMRS)**[55] — The AMRS is a five-item, patient self-rating mania scale, designed to assess the presence and/or severity of manic symptoms. The AMRS is designed to be a screening instrument, and a diagnosis can not be reliably made based upon results from this tool. All items are scored from 0 (absent) to 4 (present to a severe degree), based on increasing severity. A cutoff score of 6 or higher on the AMRS indicates a high probability of a manic or hypomanic condition (based on a sensitivity rating of 85.5 percent and a specificity rating of 87.3 percent). A score of 5 or lower is less likely to be associated with significant symptoms of mania. A score of 6 or higher may indicate a need for treatment and/or further diagnostic workup (to confirm a diagnosis of mania or hypomania).

> ▶ **The IDS-SR**[41, 56] — This is a self-report companion scale to the IDS-C described above. It includes 30 multiple-choice items, with most scored from 0 (least severe) to 3 (most severe). Completion of the IDS-SR requires approximately 15–20 minutes, and adequate reading ability. The IDS-SR is highly correlated with other self-report measures of depression (0.93 with the BDI) and with its companion, clinician-rated version (0.91 with the IDS-C).

> ▶ **The Beck Depression Inventory (BDI-2)**[57, 58] — The BDI-2 assesses depressive symptoms based on the DSM-IV criteria. The patient is asked to respond to 21 items covering specific thoughts and feelings in the areas of cognitive, affective, somatic, and vegetative symptoms of depression they have experienced within the past week. It is useful for those 13 years and older and can be administered individually or in groups in a written or oral format. It takes approximately 5–10 minutes to complete and can be scored manually or by computer, with a computer-based interpretation of the scores available. The BDI-2 is intended to be a screening tool for depression, with particular attention to items on hopelessness and suicidal ideation as the best indicators of potential suicidality.[192, 193]

Conducting a General Assessment of Psychiatric Symptoms

A trained clinician might also choose to use a general measure of psychiatric symptoms and/or personality function to assist in the diagnostic process. These measures, while they do not directly assess bipolar symptoms, can be helpful in differentiating symptoms from other disorders.

BPRS-24

The BPRS-24 is a general measure of psychiatric symptomatology, encompassing a range of symptoms and intended to assess symptom changes in psychiatric patients. This 24-item scale relies on a clinician-administered format, utilizing information gained through behavioral observation and collateral sources.[59, 60]

The initial version (BPRS-18 item) was updated to include three additional items specifically designed to capture manic phase symptoms for patients with bipolar disorder as well as increased coverage of psychiatric symptoms.[194] Items are rated on a 1- to 7-point scale of increasing severity, and the scale is available in a format that incorporates rating anchors and interview probes to enhance interrater reliability and accuracy.[195]

Good joint reliability is achievable with the BPRS, but it requires thorough training of interviewers. The BPRS has been demonstrated to provide a sensitive, though nonspecific, measure of psychiatric status change. It is correlated with other measures of general psychopathology, and specific items correlate with scales intended to measure the same symptom domain.

MMPI-2

The MMPI-2 is widely used both to assess personality characteristics that may influence response to treatment, and as a general tool to assist with diagnosis and clinical assessment.[61] It consists of 567 "true/false" questions, administered in a choice of formats, including an online administration. Results yield *T-scores* for a number of validity, basic, and clinical scales. While the MMPI-2 is a valuable part of the assessment process, particularly with a cooperative patient, understanding the results requires interpretation by a trained professional. Definitive diagnosis cannot be made solely from results on an MMPI-2, but this instrument can be helpful as part of a general diagnostic evaluation, which includes a clinical interview, observation, and other assessment approaches.

General assessment measures include:

▶ *The Brief Psychiatric Rating Scale (BPRS)*

▶ *The Minnesota Multiphasic Personality Inventory – 2nd Edition (MMPI-2)*

▶ *The Millon Clinical Multiaxial Inventory (MCMI-III)*

T-scores — standardized scores based on 0 to 100, with 50 as a mean

MCMI-III

The MCMI-III was developed to assess clinical personality styles and major clinical syndromes in accordance with Millon's theories of personality and psychopathology as well as DSM-IV categories.[62] It consists of 175 "true/false" items, scored across 24 scales.

Concerns about this instrument include the overlap between scales and the use of base rates in defining cutoff scores for scale interpretation. Individual items can count toward more than one scale, resulting in artificially high correlations between subscales. Additionally, the use of base rates may be inappropriate when the person taking the test is significantly different from those included in the standardization sample.

The scale is better at identifying personality and psychopathology according to Millon's theoretical model, and less consistent in agreement with DSM-IV diagnostic categories.

Appendix C:
Life Chart Sample

The Life Chart provides a structure to help patients monitor their moods on a daily basis with both a daily and monthly log for patient and clinician to use to review treatment response. The patient completes the log at the end of each day (prior to taking evening medication), recording information about:

A full copy of the Life Chart is available from the Depression Bipolar Support Alliance (DBSA) at www.dbsalliance.org.

▶ Medications taken

▶ Number of hours of sleep from the previous night

▶ Overall mood for the day according to a scale given (If experiencing sudden, distinct, or significant mood changes within the day, patients enter the highest and lowest mood values reached.)

▶ The number of mood changes over the course of the day

▶ The severity of mood episodes rated according to level of functional impairment

▶ Whether or not the patient is having a menstrual period (if applicable)

▶ Significant events each day in terms of life events, side effects, and coexisting symptoms

A copy of the Life Chart log follows on pages 90–91.

MONTH _____

YOUR PRESCRIPTION			1	2	3	4	5	6	7	8	9	10	11	12	13
MEDICATION NAME	DAILY DOSE	# OF PILLS PER DAY	T	O	T	A	L		N	U	M	B	E	R	

RECORD HOURS OF NIGHTTIME SLEEP __ __ __ __ __ __ __ __ __ __ __ __ __

M A N I A

DYSPHORIC MANIA (✔)IF YES		__ __ __ __ __ __ __ __ __ __ __ __ __
SEVERE	Essentially incapacitated or **HOSPITALIZED**	○○○○○○○○○○○○○
HIGH MODERATE	GREAT difficulty with goal-oriented activity	○○○○○○○○○○○○○
LOW MODERATE	SOME difficulty with goal-oriented activity	○○○○○○○○○○○○○
MILD	More energized & productive; usual routine not affected much	○○○○○○○○○○○○○
STABLE		○○○○○○○○○○○○○

D E P R E S S I O N

MILD	Usual routine not affected much	○○○○○○○○○○○○○
LOW MODERATE	Functioning with SOME effort	○○○○○○○○○○○○○
HIGH MODERATE	Functioning with GREAT effort	○○○○○○○○○○○○○
SEVERE	Essentially incapacitated or **HOSPITALIZED**	○○○○○○○○○○○○○

MOOD (0 - 100) 0 •••••••••••••50•••••••••••••100
Most depressed ever   Balanced   Most manic (activated) ever __ __ __ __ __ __ __ __ __ __ __ __ __

NUMBER OF MOOD CHANGES / DAY __ __ __ __ __ __ __ __ __ __ __ __ __

MENSTRUAL PERIOD (✔)IF YES __ __ __ __ __ __ __ __ __ __ __ __ __

1	2	3	4	5	6	7	8	9	10	11	12	13

YEAR _____

14	15	16	17	18	19	20	21	22	23	24	25	26	27	28	29	30	31

O F   P I L L S   T A K E N   P E R   D A Y

14	15	16	17	18	19	20	21	22	23	24	25	26	27	28	29	30	31

Glossary

A

abnormal grief — acute grief persisting beyond the typical two to four months that may contribute to depressive symptoms or exacerbate a bipolar depressive episode

absolute starting dose — amount of medication given when the patient first takes it

active listening — a way of listening that focuses entirely on what the other person is saying and confirms understanding of both the message content and the emotions and feelings underlying the message to ensure accurate understanding

add-on treatment — the addition of a new medication to already ongoing treatment

affect — the conscious subjective aspect of an emotion considered apart from bodily changes

algorithms — an organized, often specific set of recommendations that are evidence-based, often informed by expert consensus opinion when there are inadequate studies to inform treatment decisions

amygdala — one of the basal ganglia that is part of the limbic system and believed to be involved in impulsivity and other functions

assertive communication techniques — these techniques help patients honestly express opinions, feelings, attitudes, and rights (without undue anxiety) in a way that doesn't infringe on the rights of others

attributional style — one's tendencies in making causal explanations about a variety of intra- and interpersonal events in their lives

atypical antipsychotics — the class of antipsychotic medications with less extra-pyramidal, side-effects

atypical features — mood reactivity and at least two of the following: increased appetite or weight gain, excessive sleep, the sensation that your limbs are too heavy to move, and a long-standing pattern of sensitivity to perceived interpersonal rejection

B

behavioral rehearsal — rehearsing new responses to problematic situations

C

catatonic features — clinical features characterized by marked psychomotor disturbance that may involve immobility, excessive motor activity, extreme negativism, inability or refusal to speak, peculiar voluntary movements or speech

circadian rhythms — the daily regulation of sleep-wake cycles and activity-to-activity patterns

cotransmitters — two molecules released from the same synapse that act on an adjacent neuron, both of which are physiologically active

crossover design — a type of clinical study where patients are randomized to one treatment arm, then at some point during the study will be "crossed over" to receive the other treatment option

93

D

delusions — false, fixed, odd, or unusual beliefs about external reality that are not ordinarily accepted by other members of the person's culture or subculture, yet are firmly sustained despite clear evidence to the contrary.

depression — a mood state characterized by sadness or irritability, low energy, thoughts of death and suicide, and lack of interest in previously enjoyed activities

derailment — quality of speech characterized by loose associations or an inability to stay on topic; sequential connection between ideas; which are difficult or impossible to follow because the person wanders to relatively or totally unrelated subjects

dopamine — a neurotransmitter in the central nervous system that affects the synthesis of epinephrine

dysphoric hypomania — a mood state characterized by increased energy and symptoms of depression that do not meet full criteria for depression

epileptic seizure — an uncontrolled discharge of brain cells that spread throughout the brain, causing seizures with associated brief loss of consciousness and bladder control or aberrant excitable neural activity that stays localized (e.g., isolated limb movements, temporary blindness)

E

epileptic seizure — an uncontrolled discharge of brain cells

euthymia — normal range of mood, no evidence of mania, hypomania, or depression

evidence-based studies — medication information gained through placebo-controlled, double-blind studies (where neither the patient nor physician know who receives the "active" pill with medication versus the "sugar" pill)

executive functions — those functions of the brain carried out by the prefrontal and frontal cortex: managing stimuli, marshaling appropriate responses, and modulating impulses, which are all disrupted in the manic state

expressed emotion — critical, hostile, and overemotional communication patterns

G

genetic-laden — families that have multiple members with Bipolar Disorder or depression

goal-directed behavior — behavior directed towards accomplishing a specific task(s)

grandiosity — exaggerated belief or claims of one's importance or identity; manifested as delusions of great wealth, power, or fame when of psychotic proportions

H

habitus — body build, can refer to weight impact of medications

hallucinations — sensory perceptions (seeing, hearing, feeling, and smelling) in the absence of an outside stimulus

hippocampus — an important part of the limbic system involved in working memory and other functions

hormone receptors — a group of molecules that have diverse function throughout the brain and the body (e.g., steroid or estrogen receptors)

hypomania — a mood state characterized by increased energy, excitement, and feelings of euphoria that do not meet the diagnostic criteria for a full manic episode

I

impulsivity — taking action with limited thought to consequences

insight — understanding or awareness of one's mental or emotional condition

interitem reliability — degree to which scores on individual items agree with each other; an estimate of the extent to which the instrument is measuring a single construct.

interrater reliability — degree that different raters agree on a diagnosis based on the use of the instrument

M

maintenance treatment — an ongoing treatment believed to prevent or minimize the development of new episodes of mania, depression, or mixed states

major neurochemical receptor groups — neurotransmitter substances believed important in the normal and abnormal brain functioning

mania — a mood state characterized by an elevated or irritable mood, decreased sleep, high energy, impulsive behavior, and increased goal-directed behavior

melancholic features — loss of interest or pleasure in all, or almost all activities, and lack of reactivity to usually pleasurable stimuli.

mixed episodes — periods during which symptoms of a manic and a depressive episode are present at the same time.

N

neuropeptides — brain chemicals or medications that either decreases cell death and/or increases the birth of new brain cells (i.e., neurogenesis)

neuroprotective effect — the function of a brain chemical or medication to either decrease cell death and/or increase the birth of new brain cells (i.e., neurogenesis)

neurotransmitter — a chemical in the brain that transmits information between the nerve cells

neurotrophins — a class of molecules that triggers changes in the second messenger system(s, increasing cell survival and new cell growth

P

paranormal phenomena — altered perceptions experienced by the patient but not those around them, [e.g., hearing voices (auditory hallucinations), smelling burning rubber (olfactory hallucinations), etc.] as well as déjà vu, the sense of having already experienced what is now happening

PET imaging — technology that uses positron-labeled molecules and an oxygen blood flow tracer to develop images of brain activity versus the structural images provided by MRI

prodromal — precursor to a full episode, or less than criteria for a full-blown episode; subsyndromal symptoms

psychoeducational package — a treatment approach that includes multiple methods for educating the patient, such as: written, visual, and interactive materials to facilitate education about the disorder and treatment

psychosis —extreme impairment of a person's ability to think clearly, perceive things accurately, respond emotionally, communicate effectively, understand reality, and behave appropriately

psychotic — extreme impairment of a person's ability to think clearly, perceive things accurately, respond emotionally, communicate effectively, understand reality, and behave appropriately

R

rapid cycling — four or more manic, hypomanic, or depressive episodes in any 12-month period

rate of initial titration — the rate by which a medication is increased to what is believed to be a minimum effective dose

role-playing — helping their friend or family member acquire new communication skills by having them act out conversations in session

S

seasonal pattern — onset and remission of mood episodes occur at characteristic times of the year

sensitivity — the degree to which the instrument correctly identifies patients that do have the disorder

serotonin — a neurotransmitter from the indoleamine group that affects central nervous system functioning

somatization — multiple physical complaints involving any body system

specificity — the degree to which the instrument correctly identifies patients that do not have the disorder

specifiers — DSM-IV-defined categories for specific symptoms that may occur with bipolar disorder, such as psychotic or atypical symptoms

SPECT imaging — a single photon emission where image intensity is directly correlated to cerebral perfusion or blood flow, which is believed to be related to brain functional activity

T

T-scores — standardized scores based on 0 to 100, with 50 as a mean

tangentiality — speech characterized by giving unrelated answers to direct questions and frequently changing the topic

temporal lobe — a large lobe of each cerebral hemisphere that is in front of the occipital lobe and is believed involved in memory, mood regulation, and impulsivity

V

vagal nerve stimulation — an FDA-approved treatment for refractory epilepsy and depression now being explored for bipolar disorder

References

1. Diagnostic and Statistical Manual: Mental Disorders. Washington, DC: American Psychiatric Association; 1952

2. Goodwin FK, Jamison KR. Manic Depressive Illness. New York, NY: Oxford University Press Inc; 1990

3. Faedda GL, Baldessarini RJ, Suppes T, Tondo L, Becker I, Lipschitz DS. Pediatric onset bipolar disorder: A neglected clinical and public health problem. *Harv Rev Psychiatry* 1995;3:171-195

4. Hirschfeld RM, Lewis L, Vornik LA. Perceptions and impact of bipolar disorder: how far have we really come? Results of the national depressive and manic-depressive association 2000 survey of individuals with bipolar disorder. *J Clin Psychiatry* 2003;64(2):161-174

5. Suppes T, Leverich GS, Keck PE, Nolen WA, Denicoff KD, Altshuler LL, McElroy SL, Rush AJ, Kupka R, Frye MA, Bickel M, Post RM. The Stanley Foundation Bipolar Treatment Outcome Network. II. Demographics and illness characteristics of the first 261 patients. *J Affect Disord* 2001;67(1-3):45-59

6. Swann AC, Bowden CL, Morris D, Calabrese JR, Petty F, Small J, Dilsaver SC, Davis JM. Depression during mania. Treatment response to lithium or divalproex. *Arch Gen Psychiatry* 1997;54(1):37-42

7. Cassano GB, Frank E, Miniati M, Rucci P, Fagiolini A, Pini S, Shear MK, Maser JD. Conceptual underpinnings and empirical support for the mood spectrum. *Psychiatr Clin North Am.* 2002; 25(4):699-712.

8. Angst J. The emerging epidemiology of hypomania and bipolar II disorder. *J Affect Disord.* 1998; 50(2-3):143-51.

9. Akiskal HS, Pinto O. The evolving bipolar spectrum. Prototypes I, II, III, and IV. *Psychiatr Clin North Am.* 1999; 22(3):517-34, vii.

10. Goldberg JF, Harrow M, Grossman LS. Course and outcome in bipolar affective disorder: a longitudinal follow-up study. *Am J Psychiatry* 1995;152(3):379-384

11. Gitlin MJ, Swendsen J, Heller TL, Hammen C. Relapse and impairment in bipolar disorder. *Am J Psychiatry* 1995;152:1635-1640

12. Coryell W, Scheftner W, Keller M, Endicott J, Maser J, Klerman GL. The enduring psychosocial consequences of mania and depression. *Am J Psychiatry* 1993;150:720-727

13. Tohen M, Hennen J, Zarate CM Jr, Baldessarini RJ, Strakowski SM, Stoll AL, Faedda GL, Suppes T, Gebre-Medhin P, Cohen BM. Two-year syndromal and functional recovery in 219 cases of first-episode major affective disorder with psychotic features. *Am J Psychiatry* 2000;157(2):220-228

14. Cassano GB, Pini S, Saettoni M, Dell'Osso L. Multiple anxiety disorder comorbidity in patients with mood spectrum disorders with psychotic features. *Am J Psychiatry* 1999;156(3):474-476

15. McElroy S, Altshuler L, Suppes T, Keck P, Frye M, Denicoff K, Nolen W, Kupka R, Leverich G, Rochussen J, Rush AJ, Post R. Axis I psychiatric comorbidity and its relationship to historical illness variables in 288 patients with bipolar disorder. *Am J Psychiatry* 2001;158:3

16. Frye MA, Altshuler LL, McElroy SL, Suppes T, Keck PE, Denicoff K, Nolen WA, Kupka R, Leverich GS, Pollio C, Grunze H, Walden J, Post RM. Gender differences in prevalence, risk, and clinical correlates of alcoholism comorbidity in bipolar disorder. *Am J Psychiatry* 2003;160(5):883-889

17. Regier DA, Farmer ME, Rae DS, Locke BZ, Keith SJ, Judd LL, Goodwin FK. Comorbidity of mental disorders with alcohol and other drug abuse. Results from the Epidemiologic Catchment Area (ECA) Study. *JAMA* 1990;264(19):2511-2518

18. Goldberg JF, Garno JL, Leon AC, Kocsis JH, Portera L. A history of substance abuse complicates remission from acute mania in bipolar disorder. *J Clin Psychiatry* 1999;60(11):733-740

19. Strakowski SM, DelBello MP, Fleck DE, Arndt S. The impact of substance abuse on the course of bipolar disorder. *Biol Psychiatry* 2000;48(6):477-485

20. Diagnostic and Statistical Manual of Mental Disorders: Fourth Edition Text Revision DSM-IV (TR). Washington, DC: American Psychiatric Association; 2000

21. Dilsaver SC, Chen YW, Swann AC, Shoaib AM, Krajewski KJ. Suicidality in patients with pure and depressive mania. *Am J Psychiatry* 1994;151:1312-1315

22. Strakowski SM, McElroy SL, Keck PE Jr, West SA. Suicidality among patients with mixed and manic bipolar disorder. *Am J Psychiatry* 1996,153:674-676

23. Akiskal HS. The prevalent clinical spectrum of bipolar disorders: beyond DSM-IV. *J Clin Psychopharmacol* 1996;16(suppl 1):4S-14S

24. Grigoroiu-Serbanescu M, Nothen M, Propping P, Poustka F, Magureanu S, Vasilescu R, Marinescu E, Ardelean V. Clinical evidence for genomic imprinting in bipolar I disorder. *Acta Psychiatr Scand* 1995;92:365-370

25. Grigoroiu-Serbanescu M, Wickramaratne PJ, Hodge SE, Milea S, Mihailescu R. Genetic anticipation and imprinting in bipolar I illness. *Br J Psychiatry* 1997;170:162-166

26. Benazzi F. Depression with DSM-IV atypical features: a marker for Bipolar II disorder. *Eur Arch Psychiatry Clin Neurosci* 2000;250:53-55

27. Bowden CL. Strategies to reduce misdiagnosis of Bipolar depression. *Psychiatr Serv* 2001;52(1):51-55

28. Suppes T, Mintz, J, McElroy SL, Altshuler LL, Kupka RW, Frye MA, Keck PE Jr, Nolen WA, Leverich GS, Grunze H, Rush AJ, Post RM. Mixed hypomania in 908 patients with bipolar disorder evaluated prospectively in the Stanley Bipolar Treatment Network: A gender-specific phenomenon. *Archives of General Psychiatry* 2005; In press.

29. Solomon DA, Keitner GI, Miller IW, Shea MT, Keller. MB Course of ill-ness and maintenance treatments for patients with Bipolar Disorder. *J Clin Psychiatry* 1995;56(1):5-13

30. Ananth J, Wohl M, Ranganath V, Beshay M. Rapid cycling patients: conceptual and etiological factors. *Neuropsychobiology* 1993;27(4):193-198

31. Walden J, Normann C, Langosch J, Berger M, Grunze H. Differential treatment of Bipolar Disorder with old and new antiepileptic drugs. *Neuropsychobiology* 1998;38(3):181-184

32. Fujiwara Y, Honda T, Tanaka Y, Aoki S, Kuroda S. Comparison of early- and late-onset rapid cycling affective disorders: clinical course and response to pharmacotherapy. *J Clin Psychopharmacol* 1998;18(4):282-288

33. Post RM, Ketter TA, Pazzaglia PJ, Denicoff K, George MS, Callahan A, Leverich G, Frye M. Rational polypharmacy in the Bipolar affective disorders. *Epilepsy Res Suppl* 1996;11:153-180

34. Calabrese JR, Woyshville MJ. A medication algorithm for treatment of Bipolar rapid cycling? *J Clin Psychiatry* 1995a;56 Suppl 3:11-18

35. Calabrese JR, Woyshville MJ. Lithium therapy: limitations and alternatives in the treatment of Bipolar Disorders. *Ann Clin Psychiatry* 1995b;7(2):103-112

36. Endicott J, Spitzer RL. A diagnostic interview: the schedule for affective disorders and schizophrenia. *Arch Gen Psychiatry* 1978;35(7):837-844

37. Robins LN, Marcus L, Reich W, Cunningham R, Gallagher T. Diagnostic Interview Schedule, Version IV. St. Louis, MO, Department of Psychiatry, Washington School of Medicine, 1996

38. First MB, Spitzer RL, Gibbon M, Williams JBW. Structured Clinical Interview for DSM-IV – Clinician Version (SCID-CV) (User's Guide and Interview). Washington D.C., American Psychiatric Press, 1997

39. Young RC, Biggs JT, Ziegler BE, Mayer DA. A rating scale for mania: reliability, validity and sensitivity. *Br J Psychiatry* 1978;133:429-435

40. Altman EG, Hedeker DR, Janicak PG, Peterson JL, Davis JM. The Clinician-Administered Rating Scale for Mania (CARS-M): development, reliability, and validity. *Biol Psychiatry* 1994;36(2):124-134

41. Rush AJ, Giles DE, Schlesser MA, Fulton CL, Weissenburger J, Burns C. The Inventory for Depressive Symptomatology (IDS): preliminary findings. *Psychiatry Res* 1986;18(1):65-87

42. Hamilton M. A rating scale for depression. *J Neurol Neurosurg Psychiatry* 1960;23:56-62

43. Hamilton M. Development of a rating scale for primary depressive illness. *Br J Soc Clin Psychol* 1967;6:278-296

44. Williams JBW. A structured interview guide for the Hamilton Depression Rating Scale. *Arch Gen Psychiatry* 1988;45:742-747

45. Montgomery SA, Äsberg M. A new depression scale designed to be sensitive to change. *Br J Psychiatry* 1979;134:382-389

46. Kearns NP, Cruickshank CA, McGuigan KJ, Riley SA, Shaw SP, Snaith RP. A comparison of depression rating scales. *Br J Psychiatry* 1982;141:45-49

47. Davidson J, Turnbull CD, Strickland R, Miller R, Graves K. The Montgomery-Äsberg Depression Scale: reliability and validity. *Acta Psychiatr Scand* 1986; 73:544-548

48. Denicoff KD, Leverich GS, Nolen WA, Rush AJ, McElroy SL, Keck PE Jr, Suppes T, Altshuler LL, Kupka R, Frye MA, Hatef J, Brotman MA, Post RM: Validation of the prospective NIMH-Life-Chart Method (NIMH-LCM ™-p) for longitudinal assessment of Bipolar illness. *Psychol Med* 2000;30:1391-1397

49. Leverich GS, Post RM. Life charting of affective disorders. *CNS Spectrums* 1998;3(5):21-37

50. Post RM, Roy-Byrne PP, Uhde TW. Graphic representation of the life course of illness in patients with affective disorder. *Am J Psychiatry* 1988;145(7):844-848

51. Bauer MS, Crits-Christoph P, Ball WA, Dewees E, McAllister T, Alahi P, Cacciola J, Whybrow PC. Independent assessment of manic and depressive symptoms by self-rating. Scale characteristics and implications for the study of mania. *Arch Gen Psychiatry* 1991;48(9):807-812

52. Hirschfeld RMA, Williams JBW, Spitzer RL, Calabrese JR, Flynn L, Keck PE Jr, Lewis L, McElroy SL, Post RM, Rapport DJ, Russell JM, Sachs GS, Zajecka J: Development and validation of a screening instrument for Bipolar spectrum disorder: the Mood Disorder Questionnaire. *Am J Psychiatry* 2000;157:1873–1875

53. Hirschfeld RM, Holzer C, Calabrese JR, Weissman M, Reed M, Davies M, Frye MA, Keck PE, McElroy S, Lewis L, Tierce J, Wagner KD, Hazard E. Validity of the mood disorder questionnaire: a general population study. *Am J Psychiatry* 2003;160:178–180

54. Hirschfeld R. and Compact Clinicals (2005). Mood Disorder Questionnaire-Expanded. Kansas City, Missouri: Compact Clinicals.

55. Altman EG, Hedeker D, Peterson JL, Davis JM. The Altman Self-Rating Mania Scale. *Biol Psychiatry* 1997;42:948-955

56. Rush AJ, Gullion CM, Basco MR, Jarrett RB, Trivedi MH. The inventory of depressive symptomatology (IDS): Psychometric properties. *Psychol Med* 1996;26:477-486

57. Beck AT, Steer RA, Brown GK. Beck Depression Inventory – Second Edition Manual. San Antonio: TX, Psychological Corporation, Harcourt Brace, 1986

58. Beck AT, Steer RA, Garbin MG. Psychometric properties of the Beck Depression Inventory: twenty-five years of evaluation. *Clin Psychol Rev* 1988;8:77-100

59. Overall JE, Gorham DR. Introduction - the Brief Psychiatric Rating Scale (BPRS): Recent developments in ascertainment and scaling. *Psychopharmacol Bull* 1988;24:97-99

60. Ventura J, Nuechterlein KH, Subotnik K, Gilbert E. Symptom dimension in recent-onset schizophrenia: The 24-item expanded BPRS. International Congress on Schizophrenia Research, 1995

61. Butcher JN, Dahlstrom WG, Graham JR, Tellegen A, Kaemmer B. Minnesota Multiphasic Personality Inventory-2 (MMPI-2): Manual for Administration and Scoring. Minneapolis, MN, University of Minnesota Press, 1989

62. Millon T, Davis R, Millon C. MCMI-III Manual, 2nd Edition. Minneapolis, MN, National Computer Systems, 1997

63. Beck AT, Steer RA, Kovacs M, Garrison B. Hopelessness and eventual suicide: a 10-year prospective study of patients hospitalized with suicidal ideation. *Am J Psychiatry*. 1985 May;142(5):559-63.

64. Beck AT, Brown G, Berchick RJ, Stewart BL, Steer RA. Relationship between hopelessness and ultimate suicide: a replication with psychiatric outpatients. *Am J Psychiatry*. 1990 Feb;147(2):190-5.

65. Kowatch RA, Fristad M, Birmaher B, Wagner KD, Findling RL, Hellander M; Child Psychiatric Workgroup on Bipolar Disorder. Treatment guidelines for children and adolescents with bipolar disorder. *J Am Acad Child Adolesc Psychiatry*. 2005 Mar;44(3):213-35.

66. Faraone SV, Glatt SJ, Tsuang MT. The genetics of pediatric-onset Bipolar Disorder. *Biol Psychiatry* 2003a;53:970-977

67. Faraone SV, Tsuang MT. Heterogeneity and the genetics of Bipolar Disorder. *Am J Med Genet* 2003b;123C:1-9

68. Smoller JW, Finn CT. Family, twin, and adoption studies of Bipolar Disorder. *Am J Med Genet* 2003;123C:48-58

69. Cade JFJ. Lithium salts in the treatment of psychotic excitement. *Medical Journal of Australia* 1949; 36:349-352.

70. Manji HK, Moore GJ, Chen G. Lithium up-regulates the cytoprotective protein Bcl-2 in the CNS in vivo: a role for neurotrophic and neuroprotective effects in manic depressive illness. *J Clin Psychiatry* 2000;61 Suppl 9:82-96

71. Physicians Desk Reference, 59th ed., Montvale, N.J.: Thompsons PDR, 2005.

72. Suppes T, Dennehy, EB, TIMA procedural manual: Bipolar disorder algorithms (2002). Dallas, TX: Bipolar Disorder Module Texas Medication Algorithm Project. (available at www.dshs.state. tx.us/mhprograms/TIMA.shtm).

73. Suppes T, Dennehy EB, Hirschfeld RMA, Altshuler LL, Bowden CL, Calabrese JR, Crismon ML, Ketter TA, Sachs G, Swann AC and the Texas Consensus Conference Panel on Medication Treatment of Bipolar Disorder. The Texas Implementation of Medication Algorithms: Update to the algorithms for treatment of bipolar I disorder. *Journal of Clinical Psychiatry*, in press.

74. Hirschfeld RMA, Bowden DL, Gitlin MJ, Keck PE, Perlis RH, Suppes T, Thase ME. Practice Guideline for the treatment of patients with Bipolar Disorder (revision). *Am J Psychiatry* 2002;159 (suppl):1-50

75. Bauer MS, Callahan AM, Jampala C, Petty F, Sajatovic M, Schaefer V, Wittlin B, Powell BJ. Clinical practice guidelines for Bipolar Disorder from the Department of Veterans Affairs. *J Clin Psychiatry* 1999;60(1):9-21

76. Keck, PE Jr, Perlis RH, Otto MW, et al. The Expert Consensus Guideline Series: Treatment of Bipolar Disorder 2004. *Postgrad Med Spec Rep* 2004;1-120

77. Grunze H. Lithium in the acute treatment of Bipolar Disorders-a stocktaking. *Eur Arch Psychiatry Clin Neurosci* 2003;253:115-119

78. Suppes T, Baldessarini RJ, Faedda GL, Tohen M. Risk of recurrence following discontinuation of lithium treatment in Bipolar Disorder. *Arch Gen Psychiatry* 1991;48:1082-1088

79. Perlis RH, Sachs GS, Lafer B, Otto MW, Faraone SV, Kane JM, Rosenbaum JF. Effect of abrupt change from standard to low serum levels of lithium: a reanalysis of double-blind lithium maintenance data. *Am J Psychiatry* 2002; 159:1155-1159

80. Bowden CL, Brugger AM, Swann AC, Calabrese JR, Janicak PG, Petty F, Dilsaver SC, Davis JM, Rush AJ, Small JG, Garza-Treviño ES, Risch SC, Goodnick PJ, Morris DD. Efficacy of divalproex vs lithium and placebo in the treatment of mania. The Depakote Mania Study Group. *JAMA* 1994;271(12):918-924

81. Pope HG Jr, McElroy SL, Keck PE Jr, Hudson JI. Valproate in the treatment of acute mania. A placebo-controlled study. *Arch Gen Psychiatry* 1991;48(1):62-68

82. Joffe H, Cohen LS, Suppes T, et al. Polycistic ovarian syndrome is associated with valproate use in bipolar women. Presented at: The 157th Meeting of the American Psychiatric Association; May 1-6, 2004; New York, NY

83. Altshuler LL, Rasgon NL, Elman S, et al. Reproductive and metabolic hormone levels in bipolar women. Presented at: The 4th European Stanley Conference on Bipolar Disorders, Aarhus, Denmark, September 23-25, 2004.

84. Isojarvi JI, Laatikainen TJ, Pakarinen AJ, et al. Polycystic ovaries and hyperandrogenism in women taking valproate for epilepsy. *N Engl J Med* 1993;329:1383-1388

85. Weisler RH, Kalali AH, Ketter TA. A multicenter, randomized, double-blind, placebo-controlled trial of extended release carbamazepine capsules as monotherapy for bipolar disorder patients with manic or mixed episodes. *J Clin Psychiatry* 2004;65:478-484

86. Weisler RH, Keck PE, Swann AC. Treatment of manic and mixed patients with carbamazepine extended release. Presented at: The 157th Meeting of the American Psychiatric Association; May 1-6, 2004; New York, NY

87. Ghaemi SN, Berv DA, Klugman J, Rosenquist KJ, Hsu DJ. Oxcarbazepine treatment of Bipolar Disorder. *J Clin Psychiatry* 2003;64:943-945

88. Suppes T, Anderson R, Dennehy D, Ozcan M, Snow D, Sureddi S. An open add-on study of oxcarbazepine versus divalproex to treat hypomanic symptoms in patients with Bipolar Disorder. Abstract presented at New Clinical Drug Evaluation Unit (NCDEU) 43rd Annual Meeting, Boca Raton, FL, May 27-30, 2003.

89. Keck PE, Jr., Marcus R, Tourkodimitris S, Ali M, Liebeskind A, Saha A, Ingenito G. A placebo-controlled, double-blind study of the efficacy and safety of aripiprazole in patients with acute bipolar mania. *Am J Psychiatry* 2003;160:1651-1658

90. Sachs GS, Sanchez R, Marcus RN, et al. Aripiprazole versus placebo in patients with an acute manic or mixed episode. Presented at: The 157th Meeting of the American Psychiatric Association; May 1-6, 2004; New York, NY

91. Suppes T, Webb A, Paul B, Carmody T, Kraemer H, Rush AJ. Clinical outcome in a randomized 1-year trial of clozapine versus treatment as usual for patients with treatment-resistant illness and a history of mania. *Am J Psychiatry* 1999;156(8):1164-1169

92. Calabrese JR, Kimmel SE, Woyshville MJ, Rapport DJ, Faust CJ, Thompson PA, Meltzer HY. Clozapine for treatment-refractory mania. *Am J Psychiatry* 1996;153:759-764

93. McElroy SL, Dessain EC, Pope HG Jr, Cole JO, Keck PE Jr, Frankenberg FR, Aizley HG, O'Brien S. Clozapine in the treatment of psychotic mood disorders, schizoaffective disorder, and schizophrenia. *J Clin Psychiatry* 1991;52(10):411-414

94. Frye MA, Ketter TA, Altshuler LL, Denicoff K, Dunn RT, Kimbrell TA, Cora-Locatelli G, Post RM. Clozapine in Bipolar Disorder: treatment implications for other atypical antipsychotics. *J Affect Disord* 1998;48(2-3):91-104

95. Tohen M, Sanger TM, McElroy SL, Tollefson GD, Chengappa KN, Daniel DG, Petty F, Centorrino F, Wang R, Grundy SL, Greaney MG, Jacobs TG, David SR, Toma V. Olanzapine versus placebo in the treatment of acute mania. Olanzapine HGEH Study Group. *Am J Psychiatry* 1999;156:702-709

96. Tohen M, Jacobs TG, Grundy SL, McElroy SL, Banov MC, Janicak PG, Sanger T, Risser R, Zhang F, Toma V, Francis J, Tollefson GD, Breier A. Efficacy of olanzapine in acute bipolar mania. *Arch Gen Psychiatry* 2000;57:841-849

97. Berk M, Ichim L, Brook S. Olanzapine compared to lithium in mania: a double-blind randomized controlled trial. *Int Clin Psychopharmacol* 1999;14(6):339-343

98. Tohen M, Ketter TA, Zarate CA, et al. Olanzapine versus divalproex sodium for the treatment of acute mania and maintenance of remission: a 47-week study. *Am J Psychiatry* 2003;160:1263-1271

99. Khanna S, Victa E. Lyons B, et al. Risperidone in the treatment of acute mania: a double-blind, placebo-controlled study of 290 patients. *Br J Psychiatry*, in press

100. Hirschfeld RM, Keck PE Jr, Kramer M, et al. Rapid antimanic effect of risperidone monotherapy: a 3-week multicenter, double-blind, placebo-controlled trial. *Am J Psychiatry* 2004;161(6):1057-1065

101. Smulevich AB, Khanna S, Eerdekens M, Karcher K, Kramer M, Grossman F. Acute and continuation risperidone monotherapy in bipolar mania: a 3-week placebo-controlled trial followed by a 9-week double-blind trial of risperidone and haloperidol. *Eur Neuropsychopharmacol.* 2005 Jan;15(1):75-84.

102. Sachs GS, Grossman F, Ghaemi SN, Okamoto A, Bowden CL. Combination of a mood stabilizer with risperidone or haloperidol for treatment of acute mania: a double-blind, placebo-controlled comparison of efficacy and safety. *Am J Psychiatry* 2002;159:1146-1154

103. Yatham LN, Grossman F, Augustyns I, Vieta E, Ravindran A. Mood stabilisers plus risperidone or placebo in the treatment of acute mania. International, double-blind, randomised controlled trial. *Br J Psychiatry* 2003;182:141-147

104. Bowden CL, Grunze H, Mullen J, Brecher M, Paulsson B, Jones M, Vagero M, Svensson K. A randomized, double-blind, placebo-controlled efficacy and safety study of quetiapine or lithium as monotherapy for mania in bipolar disorder. *J Clin Psychiatry.* 2005 Jan;66(1):111-21.

105. McIntyre R, Brecher M, Poulsson B. Quetiapine or haloperidol as monotherapy for bipolar mania – a 12-week, double-blind, randomised, parallel-group, placebo-controlled trial. *Eur Neuropsychopharmacol,* in press

106. Keck PE, Jr., Versiani M, Potkin S, West SA, Giller E, Ice K. Ziprasidone in the treatment of acute bipolar mania: a three-week, placebo-controlled, double-blind, randomized trial. *Am J Psychiatry* 2003;160(4):741-748

107. Segal S, Riesenberg RA, Ice K, et al. Ziprasidone in Mania: 21-day randomized clinical trial. Presented at: The 16th Congress European College of Neuropsychopharmacology; September 20–24, 2003; Prague, Czech Republic

108. Citrome LL, Jaffe AB. Relationship of atypical antipsychotics with development of diabetes mellitus. *Ann Pharmacother* 2003;37(12):1849-1857

109. American Diabetes Association, American Psychiatric Association, American Association of Clinical Endocrinologists, North American Association for the Study of Obesity. Consensus development conference on antipsychotic drugs and obesity and diabetes. *Diabetes Care* 2004;27(2):596-601

110. Sachs GS, Printz DJ, Kahn DA, Carpenter D, Docherty JP. The Expert Consensus Guideline Series: medication treatment of Bipolar Disorder 2000. *Postgrad Med* 2000; April:1-104

111. Suppes T, Dennehy EB, Swann AC, Bowden CL, Calabrese JR, Hirschfeld RM, Keck PE Jr, Sachs GS, Crismon ML, Toprac MG, Shon SP; Texas Consensus Conference Panel on Medication Treatment of Bipolar Disorder. Report of the Texas Consensus Conference Panel on medication treatment of Bipolar Disorder 2000. *J Clin Psychiatry* 2002;63(4):288-299

112. Dennehy EB, Suppes T. Medication algorithms for Bipolar Disorder. *J Pract Psychiatry Behav Health* 1999;5:142-152

113. Bauer M, Dopfmer S. Lithium augmentation in treatment-resistant depression: meta-analysis of placebo-controlled studies. *J Clin Psychopharmacol* 1999;19(5):427-434

114. Post RM, Leverich GS, Denicoff KD, Frye MA, Kimbrell TA, Dunn R. Alternative approaches to refractory depression in bipolar illness. *Depression Anxiety* 1997;5(4):175-189

115. Ebert D, Jaspert A, Murata H, Kaschka WP. Initial lithium augmentation improves the antidepressant effects of standard TCA treatment in non-resistant depressed patients. *Psychopharmacology* 1995;118(2):223-225

116. Fieve RR, Kumbaraci T, Dunner DL. Lithium prophylaxis of depression in bipolar I, bipolar II, and unipolar patients. *Am J Psychiatry* 1976;133(8):925-929

117. Prien RF, Caffey EM, Klett CJ. Prophylactic efficacy of lithium carbonate in manic-depressive illness. Report of the Veterans Administration and National Institute of Mental Health collaborative study group. *Arch Gen Psychiatry* 1973;28(3):337-341

118. Bowden CL, Calabrese JR, Sachs G, Yatham LN, Asghar SA, Hompland M, Montgomery P, Earl N, Smoot TM, DeVeaugh-Geiss J. A placebo-controlled 18-month trial of lamotrigine and lithium maintenance treatment in recently manic or hypomanic patients with bipolar I disorder. *Arch Gen Psychiatry* 2003;60(4):392-400

119. Calabrese JR, Bowden CL, Sachs G, Yatham LN, Behnke K, Mehtonen OP, Montgomery P, Ascher J, Paska W, Earl N, DeVeaugh-Geiss J. A placebo-controlled 18-month trial of lamotrigine and lithium maintenance treatment in recently depressed patients with bipolar I disorder. *J Clin Psychiatry* 2003;64:1013-1024

120. Goodwin FK, Fireman B, Simon GE, Hunkeler EM, Lee J, Revicki D. Suicide risk in Bipolar Disorder during treatment with lithium and divalproex. *JAMA* 2003;290:1467-1473

121. Wehr TA, Goodwin FK. Can antidepressants cause mania and worsen the course of affective illness? *Am J Psychiatry* 1987;144(11):1403-1411

122. Coryell W, Endicott J, Maser JD, Keller MB, Leon AC, Akiskal HS. Long-term stability of polarity distinctions in the affective disorders. *Am J Psychiatry* 1995;152(3):385-390

123. Altshuler LL, Post RM, Leverich GS, Mikalauskas K, Rosoff A, Ackerman L. Antidepressant-induced mania and cycle acceleration: a controversy revisited. *Am J Psychiatry* 1995;152(8):1130-1138

124. Nemeroff CB, Evans DL, Gyulai L, Sachs GS, Bowden CL, Gergel IP, Oakes R, Pitts CD. Double-blind, placebo-controlled comparison of imipramine and paroxetine in the treatment of bipolar depression. *Am J Psychiatry* 2001;158:906-912

125. Post RM. Weiss SR. Sensitization and kindling phenomena in mood, anxiety, and obsessive-compulsive disorders: the role of serotonergic mechanisms in illness progression. *Biol Psychiatry* 1998;44(3):193-206

126. Post RM, Altshuler LL, Leverich GS, et al. Switch rate on venlafaxine compared with bupropion and sertraline. Presented at: The 4th European Stanley Conference on Bipolar Disorders: September 23-25, 2004: Aarhus, Denmark

127. Post RM, Altshuler LL, Frye MA, et al. Rate of switch in bipolar patients prospectively treated with second-generation antidepressants as augmentation to mood stabilizers. *Bipolar Disord* 2001;3:259-265

128. Nolen WA, Bloemkolk D. Treatment of bipolar depression, a review of the literature and a suggestion for an algorithm. *Neuropsychobiology* 2000;42(suppl 1):11-17

129. Young LT, Joffe RT, Robb JC, MacQueen GM, Marriott M, Patelis-Siotis I. Double-blind comparison of addition of a second mood stabilizer versus an antidepressant to an initial mood stabilizer for treatment of patients with bipolar depression. *Am J Psychiatry* 2000;157(1):124-126

130. Altshuler LL, Rasgon NL, Elman S, et al. Reproductive and metabolic hormone levels in bipolar women. Presented at: The 4th European Stanley Conference on Bipolar Disorders, Aarhus, Denmark, September 23-25, 2004

131. Altshuler L, Suppes T, Black D, Nolen WA, Keck PE, Frye MA, McElroy S, Kupka R, Grunze H, Walden J, Leverich G, Denicoff K, Luckenbaugh D, Post RM. Impact of Antidepressant Discontinuation After Acute Bipolar Depression Remission on Rates of Depressive Relapse at 1-Year Follow-Up. *Am J Psychiatry* 2003;160(7):1252-1262

132. Calabrese JR, Keck PE Jr, Macfadden W, et al. A randomized, double-blind, placebo-controlled trial of quetiapine in the treatment of bipolar I or II depression. *Am J Psychiatry*, in press

133. Calabrese JR, Bowden CL, Sachs GS, Ascher JA, Monaghan E, Rudd GD. A double-blind placebo-controlled study of lamotrigine monotherapy in outpatients with bipolar I depression. Lamictal 602 Study Group. *J Clin Psychiatry* 1999;60(2):79-88

134. Frye MA, Ketter TA, Kimbrell TA, Dunn RT, Speer AM, Osuch EA, Luckenbaugh DA, Cora-Ocatelli G, Leverich GS, Post RM. A placebo-controlled study of lamotrigine and gabapentin monotherapy in refractory mood disorders. *J Clin Psychopharmacol* 2000;20(6):607-614

135. Gijsman HJ, Geddes JR, Rendell JM, et al. Antidepressants for bipolar depression: a systematic review of randomized, Controlled Trials. *Am J Psychiatry* 2004;161:1537-1547

136. Boerlin HL, Gitlin MJ, Zoellner LA, et al. Bipolar depression and antidepressant-induced mania: a naturalistic study. *J Clin Psychiatry* 1998;59(7):374-379

137. Kupfer DJ, Chengappa KN, Gelenberg AJ, et al. Citalopram as adjunctive therapy in bipolar depression. *J Clin Psychiatry* 2001;62(12):985-990

138. Vieta E, Martinez-Aran A, Goikolea JM, et al. A randomized trial comparing paroxetine and venlafaxine in the treatment of bipolar depressed patients taking mood stabilizers. *J Clin Psychiatry* 2002;63(6):508-512

139. Tohen M, Vieta E, Calabrese J, Ketter TA, Sachs G, Bowden C, Mitchell PB, Centorrino F, Risser R, Baker RW, Evans AR, Beymer K, Dube S, Tollefson GD, Breier A. Efficacy of olanzapine and olanzapine-fluoxetine combination in the treatment of bipolar I depression. *Arch Gen Psychiatry* 2003;60:1079-1088

140. Ketter TA, Post RM, Parekh PI, Worthington K. Addition of monoamine oxidase inhibitors to carbamazepine: preliminary evidence of safety and antidepressant efficacy in treatment-resistant depression. *J Clin Psychiatry* 1995;56(10):471-475

141. Thase ME, Mallinger AG, McKnight D, Himmelhoch JM. Treatment of imipramine-resistant recurrent depression, IV: A double-blind crossover study of tranylcypromine for anergic bipolar depression. *Am J Psychiatry* 1992;149(2):195-198

142. Himmelhoch JM, Thase ME, Mallinger AG, Houck P. Tranylcypromine versus imipramine in anergic bipolar depression. *Am J Psychiatry* 1991;148(7):910-916

143. Cohn JB, Collins G, Ashbrook E, Wernicke JF. A comparison of fluoxetine imipramine and placebo in patients with bipolar depressive disorder. *Int Clin Psychopharmacol* 1989;4(4):313-322

144. Sachs GS, Lafer B, Stoll AL, Banov M, Thibault AB, Tohen M, Rosenbaum JF. A double-blind trial of bupropion versus desipramine for bipolar depression. *J Clin Psychiatry* 1994;55(9):391-393

145. Ketter RA, Kalali AH, Weisler RH. A 6-month, multicenter, open-label evaluation of beaded, extended-release carbamazepine capsule monotherapy in bipolar disorder patients with manic or mixed episodes. *J Clin Psychiatry* 2004;65:668-673

146. Tohen MF, Bowden CL, Calabrese JR, et al. Olanzapine Versus Placebo for Relapse Prevention in Bipolar Disorder. Presented at: The 156th Meeting of the American Psychiatric Association; May 17-22, 2003; San Francisco, CA

147. Tohen MF, Marneros A, Bowden CL, et al. Olanzapine versus lithium in relapse prevention in bipolar disorder. Presented at: The 156th Meeting of the American Psychiatric Association; May 17-22, 2003; San Francisco, CA

148. Keck PE, Sanchez R, Marcus RN, et al. Aripiprazole for relapse prevention in bipolar disorder in a 26-week trial. Presented at: The 157th Meeting of the American Psychiatric Association; May 1-6, 2004; New York, NY

149. American Psychiatric Association. Practice guidelines for the treatment of patients with Bipolar Disorder (revision). *Am J Psychiatry* 2002;159(4 Suppl):1-50

150. Mukherjee S, Sackeim HA, Schnurr DB. Electroconvulsive therapy of acute manic episode: a review of 50 years' experience. *Am J Psychiatry* 1994;151(2):169-176

151. Small JG, Klapper MH, Kellams JJ, Miller MJ, Milstein V, Sharpley PH, Small IF. Electroconvulsive treatment compared with lithium in the management of manic states. *Arch Gen Psychiatry* 1988;45(8):727-732

152. Ernst E. Safety concerns about kava. *Lancet* 2002;359:1865

153. Otto MW, Reilly-Harrington N, Sachs GS. Psychoeducational and cognitive-behavioral strategies in the management of bipolar disorder. *J Affect Disord.* 2003 Jan:73 (1-2); 171081.

154. Gonzalez-Pinto A, Gonzalez C, Enjuto S, Fernandez de Corres B, Lopez P, Palomo J, Gutierrez M, Mosquera F, Perez de Heredia JL. Psychoeducation and cognitive-behavioral therapy in bipolar disorder: an update. *Acta Psychiatr Scand.* 2004 Feb;109(2):83-90.

155. Swartz HA, Frank E. Psychotherapy for bipolar depression: A phase specific treatment strategy? *Bipolar Disord* 2001;3:11-22

156. Callahan AM, Bauer MS. Psychosocial interventions for bipolar disorder. *Psychiatr Clin North Am.* 1999 Sep;22(3):675-88, x.

157. Scott J. Cognitive therapy of affective disorders: a review. *J Affect Disord.* 1996 Feb 12;37(1):1-11.

158. Keck PE Jr, McElroy SL, Strakowski SM, Stanton SP, Kizer DL, Balistreri TM, Bennett JA, Tugrul KC, West SA. Factors associated with pharmacologic noncompliance in patients with mania. *J Clin Psychiatry* 1996;57:292-297

159. Keck PE Jr, McElroy SL, Strakowski SM, West SA, Sax KW, Hawkins JM, Bourne ML, Haggard P. Twelve-month outcome of patients with Bipolar Disorder following hospitalization for a manic or mixed episode. *Am J Psychiatry* 1998;155:646-652

160. Johnson RE, McFarland BH. Lithium use and discontinuation in a health maintenance organization. *Am J Psychiatry* 1996;153:993-1000

161. Lingam R, Scott J. Treatment non-adherence in affective disorders. *Acta Psychiatr Scand.* 2002 Mar;105(3):164-72.

162. Frank E, Swartz HA, Kupfer DJ. Interpersonal and social rhythm therapy: managing the chaos of Bipolar Disorder. *Biol Psychiatry* 2000;48(6):593-604

163. Johnson SL, Roberts JE. Life events and Bipolar Disorder: Implications from biological theories. *Psychol Bull* 1995;117:434-449

164. Reilly-Harrington NA, Alloy LB, Fresco DM, Whitehouse WG. Cognitive styles and life events interact to predict bipolar and unipolar symptomatology. *J Abnorm Psychol* 1999;108(4):567-578

165. Johnson SL, Winett CA, Meyer B, Greenhouse WJ, Miller I: Social support and the course of Bipolar Disorder. *J Abnorm Psychol* 1999;108:558-566

166. Tohen M, Waternaux CM, Tsuang MT. Outcome in mania: A 4-year prospective follow-up of 75 patients utilizing survival analysis. *Arch Gen Psychiatry* 1990;47:1106-1111

167. Hammen C, Gitlin M, Altshuler L. Predictors of work adjustment in bipolar I patients: a naturalistic longitudinal follow-up. *J Consult Clin Psychol* 2000;68:220-225

168. Dion G, Tohen M, Anthony W, Waternaux C. Symptoms and functioning of patients with Bipolar Disorder six months after hospitalization. *Hosp Commun Psychiatry* 1988;39:652-656

169. Bauer M, McBride L. Structured Group Psychotherapy for Bipolar Disorder: The Life Goals Program. New York: Springer Publishing Company, Inc., 1996

170. Toprac MG, Rush AJ, Conner TM, Crismon ML, Dees M, Hopkins C, Rowe V, Shon SP. The Texas Medication Algorithm Project patient and family education program: a consumer-guided initiative. *J Clin Psychiatry* 2000;61:477-486

171. Colom F, Vieta E, Reinares M, Martinez-Aran A, Torrent C, Goikolea JM, Gasto C. Psychoeducation efficacy in bipolar disorders: beyond compliance enhancement. *J Clin Psychiatry.* 2003 Sep;64(9):1101-5.

172. Perry A, Tarrier N, Morriss R, McCarthy E, Limb K. Randomised controlled trial of efficacy of teaching patients with Bipolar Disorder to identify early symptoms of relapse and obtain treatment. *Br Med J* 1999;318:149-153

173. Seltzer A, Roncari I, Garfinkel P. Effect of patient education on medication compliance. *Can J Psychiatry* 1980;25:638-645

174. Peet M, Harvey NS. Lithium maintenance, 1: a standard education programme for patients. *Br J Psychiatry* 1991; 158: 197-200

175. Miklowitz DJ, Goldstein MJ. Bipolar Disorder: A Family-Focused Treatment Approach. New York: Guilford, 1997

176. Miklowitz DJ, Simoneau TL, George EL, Richards JA, Kalbag A, Sachs-Ericsson N, Suddath R. Family-focused treatment of Bipolar Disorder: 1-year effects of a psychoeducational program in conjunction with pharmacotherapy. *Biol Psychiatry* 2000;48:582-592

177. Miklowitz, DJ, George, EL, Richards, JA, Simoneau TL, Suddath, RL. A randomized study of family-focused psychoeducation and pharmacotherapy in the outpatient management of bipolar disorder. *Archives of General Psychiatry* 2003; 60: 904-912.

178. Rea MM, Tompson M, Miklowitz DJ, Goldstein MJ, Hwang S, Mintz J. Family focused treatment vs. individual treatment for Bipolar Disorder: Results of a randomized clinical trial. *J Consult Clin Psychol* 2003;71(3):482-492

179. Basco MR, Rush AJ. Cognitive-behavioral therapy for Bipolar Disorder. New York: Guilford Press, 1996

180. Cochran S. Preventing medical noncompliance in the outpatient treatment of bipolar affective disorders. *J Consult Clin Psychol* 1984;52:873-878

181. Scott J, Garland A, Moorhead S. A pilot study of cognitive therapy in Bipolar Disorders. *Psychol Med* 2001;31:459-467

182. Lam DH, Watkins ER, Hayward P, et al. A randomized controlled study of cognitive therapy for relapse prevention for bipolar affective disorder. *Arch Gen Psych* 2003;60:145-152

183. Klerman GL, Weissman MM, Rounsaville BJ, Chevron RS. Interpersonal Psychotherapy of Depression. New York, NY: Basic Books; 1984

184. Weissman MM, Markowitz J, Klerman GL. Comprehensive Guide to Interpersonal Psychotherapy. New York, NY: Basic Books; 2000

185. Frank E, Hlastala S, Ritenour A, Houck P, Tu XM, Monk TH, Mallinger AG, Kupfer DJ. Inducing lifestyle regularity in recovering Bipolar Disorder patients: Results from the maintenance therapies in Bipolar Disorder protocol. *Biol Psychiatry* 1997;41:1165-1173

186. Frank E. Interpersonal and social rhythm therapy prevents depressive symptomatology in bipolar I patients. *Bipolar Disord* 1999;1 (suppl 1):13

187. Frank E, Swartz HA, Mallinger AG, Thase ME, Weaver EV, Kupfer DJ. Adjunctive psychotherapy for Bipolar Disorder: effects of changing treatment modality. *J Abnorm Psychol* 1999;108:579-587

188. van Gent EM, Zwart FM. Psychoeducation of partners of bipolar-manic patients. *J Affect Disord*. 1991 Jan;21(1):15-8.

189. Helzer JE, Spitznagel EL, McEvoy L. The predictive validity of lay Diagnostic Interview Schedule diagnoses in the general population. A comparison with physician examiners. *Arch Gen Psychiatry* 1987;44(12):1069-1077

190. Rogers R. Diagnostic and structured interviewing: a handbook for psychologists. Odessa: FL: Psychological Assessment Resources, 1995

191. Potts MK, Daniels M, Burnam MA, Wells KB. A structured interview version of the Hamilton Depression Rating Scale: evidence of reliability and versatility of administration. *J Psychiatr Res* 1990;24(4):335-350

192. Carlson GA. Mania and ADHD: comorbidity or confusion. *J Affect Disord*. 1998 Nov;51(2):177-87.

193. Murphy LL, Impara JC, & Plake, BS (eds). (1999) Tests in print V. Lincoln, NE: University of Nebraska Press

194. Bigelow L, Murphy DL. Guidelines and Anchor Points for Modified BPRS. Unpublished manuscript, NIMH Intramural Research Program, Saint Elizabeth's Hospital, 1978

195. Essock SM, Hargreaves WA, Covell NH, Goethe J. Clozapine's effectiveness for patients in state hospitals: results from a randomized trial. *Psychopharmacol Bull* 1996;32(4):683-697

Index

We Want Your Opinion!

Comments about **Bipolar Disorder**:

_____

_____

_____

_____

_____

Other titles you would like Compact Clinicals to offer:

_____

_____

_____

_____

To be placed on our mailing list, please provide the following:

Name: _____

Address: _____

_____

_____

E-mail: _____

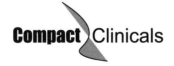

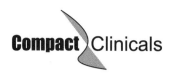

Compact Clinicals

Order in 3 easy steps:

▶ 1   Provide complete billing and shipping information

Name _____ Company_____

Profession_____ Dept./Mail Stop_____

Street Address/P.O. Box_____

City/State/Zip_____

Telephone_____ ☐ Ship to Residence   ☐ Ship to Business

▶ 2   Choose Titles

Title	Qty.	Unit Price	Total
Attention Deficit Hyperactivity Disorder *The latest assessment and treatment strategies*		$16.95	
Bipolar Disorder *The latest assessment and treatment strategies*		$16.95	
Bipolar Disorder: Treatment and Management		$18.95	
Borderline Personality Disorder *The latest assessment and treatment strategies*		$16.95	
Conduct Disorders *The latest assessment and treatment strategies*		$16.95	
Depression in Adults *The latest assessment and treatment strategies*		$16.95	
Obsessive Compulsive Disorder *The latest assessment and treatment strategies*		$16.95	
Post-Traumatic and Acute Stress Disorders *The latest assessment and treatment strategies*		$16.95	

Continuing Education credits
available for mental health professionals.
Call 1-800-408-8830 for details.

Subtotal	
Tax (Add 7.975% in MO)	
Shipping ($3.75 first book/ $1.00 per additional book)	
TOTAL	

▶ 3   Choose Payment Method

Please charge my: ☐ Visa   ☐ MasterCard   ☐ Discover   ☐ American Express   ☐ Check Enclosed

Account # __ __ __ __ — __ __ __ __ — __ __ __ __ — __ __ __ __   Exp. Date __ __ / __ __

Name on Card _____ Cardholder Signature _____

Postal Orders: Compact Clinicals, 7205 NW Waukomis Dr., Suite A, Kansas City, MO 64151

Telephone Orders: Toll Free 1-800-408-8830   **Fax Orders:** 1(816)587-7198

We Want Your Opinion!

Comments about **Bipolar Disorder**:

_____

_____

_____

_____

_____

Other titles you would like Compact Clinicals to offer:

_____

_____

_____

_____

To be placed on our mailing list, please provide the following:

Name: _____

Address: _____

_____

_____

E-mail: _____

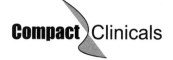

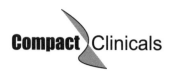

Order in 3 easy steps:

▶ 1 Provide complete billing and shipping information

Name _____ Company_____

Profession_____ Dept./Mail Stop_____

Street Address/P.O. Box_____

City/State/Zip_____

Telephone_____ ☐ Ship to Residence ☐ Ship to Business

▶ 2 Choose Titles

Title	Qty.	Unit Price	Total
Attention Deficit Hyperactivity Disorder *The latest assessment and treatment strategies*		$16.95	
Bipolar Disorder *The latest assessment and treatment strategies*		$16.95	
Bipolar Disorder: Treatment and Management		$18.95	
Borderline Personality Disorder *The latest assessment and treatment strategies*		$16.95	
Conduct Disorders *The latest assessment and treatment strategies*		$16.95	
Depression in Adults *The latest assessment and treatment strategies*		$16.95	
Obsessive Compulsive Disorder *The latest assessment and treatment strategies*		$16.95	
Post-Traumatic and Acute Stress Disorders *The latest assessment and treatment strategies*		$16.95	

Subtotal	
Tax (Add 7.975% in MO)	
Shipping ($3.75 first book/ $1.00 per additional book)	
TOTAL	

*Continuing Education credits
available for mental health professionals.
Call 1-800-408-8830 for details.*

▶ 3 Choose Payment Method

Please charge my: ☐ Visa ☐ MasterCard ☐ Discover ☐ American Express   ☐ Check Enclosed

Account # __ __ __ __ — __ __ __ __ — __ __ __ __ — __ __ __ __   Exp. Date __ __ / __ __

Name on Card _____ Cardholder Signature _____

Postal Orders: Compact Clinicals, 7205 NW Waukomis Dr., Suite A, Kansas City, MO 64151

Telephone Orders: Toll Free 1-800-408-8830   **Fax Orders:** 1(816)587-7198